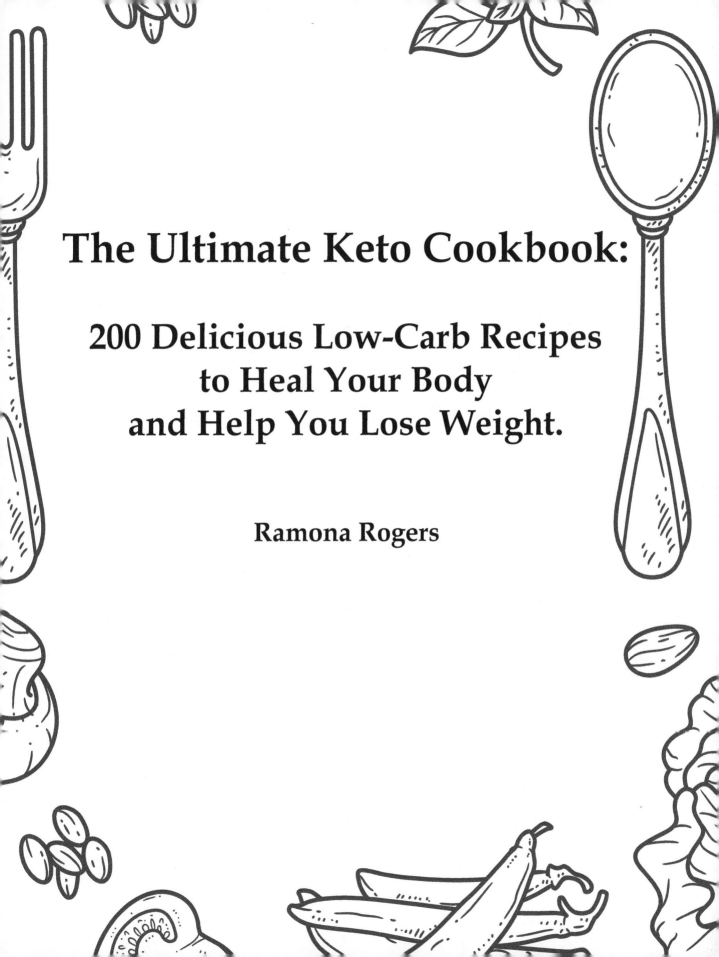

The Ultimate Keto Cookbook:

200 Delicious Low-Carb Recipes to Heal Your Body and Help You Lose Weight.

Ramona Rogers

TABLE
OF CONTENTS

Fish

Poultry

Meat

Vegetables

FISH
AND SEAFOOD

Special Fish Pie

Preparation time: 10 minutes
Cooking time: 1 hour and 10 minutes
Servings: 6

Ingredients:
1 red onion, chopped
2 salmon fillets, skinless and cut
into medium pieces
2 mackerel fillets, skinless and cut
into medium pieces
3 haddock fillets and cut into medium pieces
2 bay leaves
¼ cup ghee+ 2 tablespoons ghee
1 cauliflower head, florets separated
4 eggs
4 cloves, 1 cup whipping cream, ½ cup water
A pinch of nutmeg, ground
1 teaspoon Dijon mustard
1 cup cheddar cheese, shredded+ ½ cup cheddar cheese, shredded, Some chopped parsley
Salt and black pepper to the taste, 4 tablespoons chives, chopped

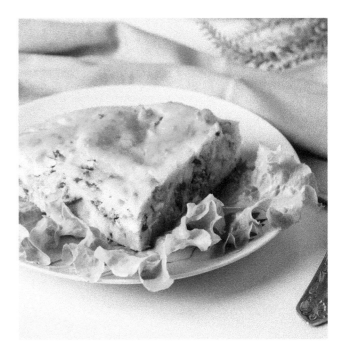

Directions:
1. Put some water in a pan, add some salt, bring to a boil over medium heat, add eggs, , cook them for 10 minutes, take off heat, drain, leave them to cool down, peel and cut them into quarters. Put water in another pot, bring to a boil, add cauliflower florets, cook for 10 minutes, drain them, transfer to your blender, add ¼ cup ghee, pulse well and transfer to a bowl.
2. Put cream and ½ cup water in a pan, add fish, toss to coat and heat up over medium heat.
3. Add onion, cloves and bay leaves, bring to a boil, reduce heat and simmer for 10 minutes.
4. Take off heat, transfer fish to a baking dish and leave aside.
5. return pan with fish sauce to heat, add nutmeg, stir and cook for 5 minutes.
6. Take off heat, discard cloves and bay leaves, add 1 cup cheddar cheese and 2 tablespoons ghee and stir well. Place egg quarters on top of the fish in the baking dish.
7. Add cream and cheese sauce over them, top with cauliflower mash, sprinkle the rest of the cheddar cheese, chives and parsley, introduce in the oven at 400 degrees F for 30 minutes.
8. Leave the pie to cool down a bit before slicing and serving.
Enjoy!

Nutrition: calories 300, fat 45, fiber 3, carbs 5, protein 26

Tasty Baked Fish

Preparation time: 10 minutes
Cooking time: 30 minutes
Servings: 4

Ingredients:
1 pound haddock
3 teaspoons water
2 tablespoons lemon juice
Salt and black pepper to the taste
2 tablespoons mayonnaise
1 teaspoon dill weed
Cooking spray
A pinch of old bay seasoning

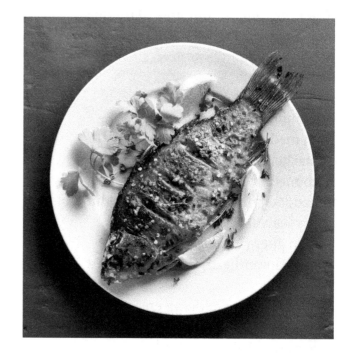

Directions:
1. Spray a baking dish with some cooking oil.
2. Add lemon juice, water and fish and toss to coat a bit.
3. Add salt, pepper, old bay seasoning and dill weed and toss again.
4. Add mayo and spread well.
5. Introduce in the oven at 350 degrees F and bake for 30 minutes.
6. Divide between plates and serve.
Enjoy!

Nutrition: calories 104, fat 12, fiber 1, carbs 0.5, protein 20

Amazing Tilapia

Preparation time: 10 minutes
Cooking time: 10 minutes
Servings: 4

Ingredients:
4 tilapia fillets, boneless
Salt and black pepper to the taste
½ cup parmesan, grated
4 tablespoons mayonnaise
¼ teaspoon basil, dried
¼ teaspoon garlic powder
2 tablespoons lemon juice
¼ cup ghee
Cooking spray
A pinch of onion powder

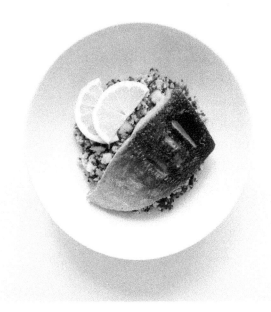

Directions:
1. Spray a baking sheet with cooking spray, place tilapia on it, season with salt and pepper, introduce in preheated broiler and cook for 3 minutes.
2. Turn fish on the other side and broil for 3 minutes more.
3. In a bowl, mix parmesan with mayo, basil, garlic, lemon juice, onion powder and ghee and stir well.
4. Add fish to this mix, toss to coat well, place on baking sheet again and broil for 3 minutes more.
5. Transfer to plates and serve.
Enjoy!

Nutrition: calorics 175, fat 10, fibcr 0, carbs 2, protcin 17

Amazing Trout And Special Sauce

Preparation time: 10 minutes
Cooking time: 10 minutes
Servings: 1

Ingredients:
1 big trout fillet
Salt and black pepper to the taste
1 tablespoon olive oil
1 tablespoon ghee
Zest and juice from 1 orange
A handful parsley, chopped
½ cup pecans, chopped

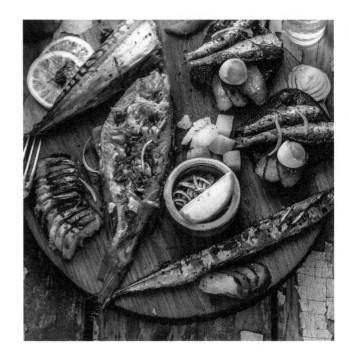

Directions:
1. Heat up a pan with the oil over medium high heat, add the fish fillet, season with salt and pepper, cook for 4 minutes on each side, transfer to a plate and keep warm for now.
2. Heat up the same pan with the ghee over medium heat, add pecans, stir and toast for 1 minutes.
3. Add orange juice and zest, some salt and pepper and chopped parsley, stir, cook for 1 minute and pour over fish fillet.
4. Serve right away.
Enjoy!

Nutrition: calories 200, fat 10, fiber 2, carbs 1, protein 14

Wonderful Trout And Ghee Sauce

Preparation time: 10 minutes
Cooking time: 10 minutes
Servings: 4

Ingredients:
4 trout fillets
Salt and black pepper to the taste
3 teaspoons lemon zest, grated
3 tablespoons chives, chopped
6 tablespoons ghee
2 tablespoons olive oil
2 teaspoons lemon juice

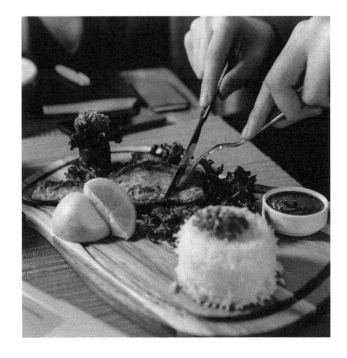

Directions:
1. Season trout with salt and pepper, drizzle the olive oil and massage a bit.
2. Heat up your kitchen grill over medium high heat, add fish fillets, cook for 4 minutes, flip and cook for 4 minutes more.
3. Meanwhile, heat up a pan with the ghee over medium heat, add salt, pepper, chives, lemon juice and zest and stir well.
4. Divide fish fillets on plates, drizzle the ghee sauce over them and serve.
Enjoy!

Nutrition: calories 320, fat 12, fiber 1, carbs 2, protein 24

Roasted Salmon

Preparation time: 10 minutes
Cooking time: 12 minutes
Servings: 4

Ingredients:
2 tablespoons ghee, soft
1 and ¼ pound salmon fillet
2 ounces Kimchi, finely chopped
Salt and black pepper to the taste

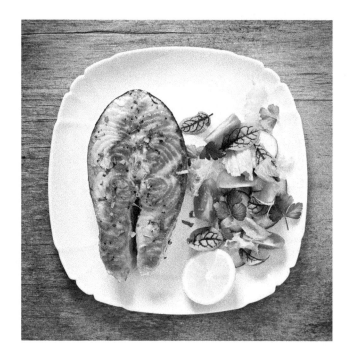

Directions:
1. In your food processor, mix ghee with Kimchi and blend well.
2. Rub salmon with salt, pepper and Kimchi mix and place into a baking dish.
3. Introduce in the oven at 425 degrees F and bake for 15 minutes.
4. Divide between plates and serve with a side salad.
Enjoy!

Nutrition: calories 200, fat 12, fiber 0, carbs 3, protein 21

Delicious Salmon Meatballs

Preparation time: 10 minutes
Cooking time: 30 minutes
Servings: 4

Ingredients:
2 tablespoons ghee
2 garlic cloves, minced
1/3 cup onion, chopped
1 pound wild salmon, boneless and minced
¼ cup chives, chopped
1 egg
2 tablespoons Dijon mustard
1 tablespoon coconut flour
Salt and black pepper to the taste
For the sauce:
4 garlic cloves, minced
2 tablespoons ghee
2 tablespoons Dijon mustard
Juice and zest of 1 lemon
2 cups coconut cream, 2 tablespoons chives, chopped

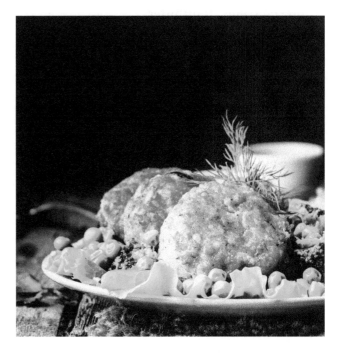

Directions:
1. Heat up a pan with 2 tablespoons ghee over medium heat, add onion and 2 garlic cloves, stir, cook for 3 minutes and transfer to a bowl.
2. In another bowl, mix onion and garlic with salmon, chives, coconut flour, salt, pepper, 2 tablespoons mustard and egg and stir well.
3. Shape meatballs from the salmon mix, place on a baking sheet, introduce in the oven at 350 degrees F and bake for 25 minutes.
4. Meanwhile, heat up a pan with 2 tablespoons ghee over medium heat, add 4 garlic cloves, stir and cook for 1 minute.
5. Add coconut cream, 2 tablespoons Dijon mustard, lemon juice and zest and chives, stir and cook for 3 minutes.
6. Take salmon meatballs out of the oven, drop them into the Dijon sauce, toss, cook for 1 minute and take off heat.
7. Divide into bowls and serve.
Enjoy!

Nutrition: calories 171, fat 5, fiber 1, carbs 6, protein 23

Salmon With Caper Sauce

Preparation time: 10 minutes
Cooking time: 20 minutes
Servings: 3

Ingredients:
3 salmon fillets
Salt and black pepper to the taste
1 tablespoon olive oil
1 tablespoon Italian seasoning
2 tablespoons capers
3 tablespoons lemon juice
4 garlic cloves, minced
2 tablespoons ghee

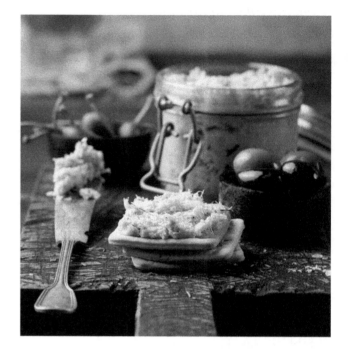

Directions:
1. Heat up a pan with the olive oil over medium heat, add fish fillets skin side up, season them with salt, pepper and Italian seasoning, cook for 2 minutes, flip and cook for 2 more minutes, take off heat, cover pan and leave aside for 15 minutes.
2. Transfer fish to a plate and leave them aside.
3. Heat up the same pan over medium heat, add capers, lemon juice and garlic, stir and cook for 2 minutes.
4. Take the pan off the heat, add ghee and stir very well.
5. Return fish to pan and toss to coat with the sauce.
6. Divide between plates and serve.
Enjoy!

Nutrition: calories 245, fat 12, fiber 1, carbs 3, protein 23

Simple Grilled Oysters

!

Preparation time: 10 minutes
Cooking time: 10 minutes
Servings: 3

Ingredients:
6 big oysters, shucked
3 garlic cloves, minced
1 lemon cut in wedges
1 tablespoon parsley
A pinch of sweet paprika
2 tablespoons melted ghee

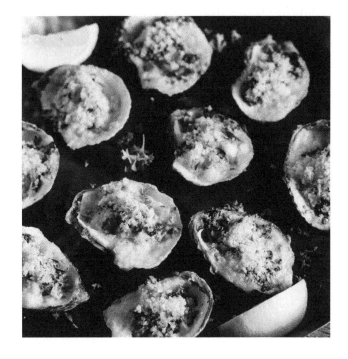

Directions:
1. Top each oyster with melted ghee, parsley, paprika and ghee.
2. Place them on preheated grill over medium high heat and cook for 8 minutes.
3. Serve them with lemon wedges on the side.
Enjoy!

Nutrition: calories 60, fat 1, fiber 0, carbs 0.6, protein 1

Baked Halibut

Preparation time: 10 minutes
Cooking time: 10 minutes
Servings: 4

Ingredients
:½ cup parmesan, grated
¼ cup ghee
¼ cup mayonnaise
2 tablespoons green onions, chopped
6 garlic cloves, minced
A dash of Tabasco sauce
4 halibut fillets
Salt and black pepper to the taste
Juice of ½ lemon

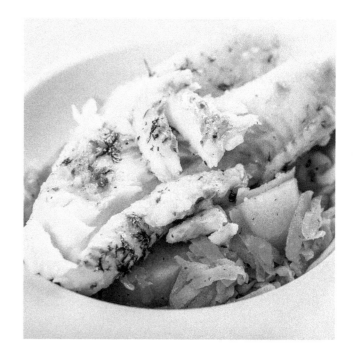

Directions:
1. Season halibut with salt, pepper and some of the lemon juice, place in a baking dish and cook in the oven at 450 degrees F for 6 minutes.
2. Meanwhile, heat up a pan with the ghee over medium heat, add parmesan, mayo, green onions, Tabasco sauce, garlic and the
rest of the lemon juice and stir well.
3. Take fish out of the oven, drizzle parmesan sauce all over, turn oven to broil and broil your fish for 3 minutes.
4. Divide between plates and serve.
Enjoy!

Nutrition: calories 240, fat 12, fiber 1, carbs 5, protein 23

Crusted Salmon

Preparation time: 10 minutes
Cooking time: 15 minutes
Servings: 4

Ingredients:
3 garlic cloves, minced
2 pounds salmon fillet
Salt and black pepper to the taste
½ cup parmesan, grated
¼ cup parsley, chopped

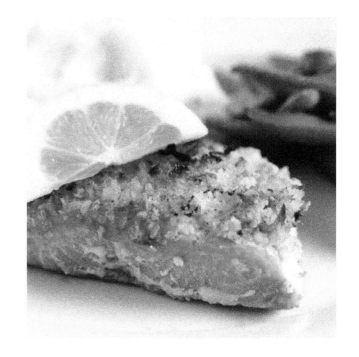

Directions:
1. Place salmon on a lined baking sheet, season with salt and pepper, cover with a parchment paper, introduce in the oven at 425 degrees F and bake for 10 minutes.
2. Take fish out of the oven, sprinkle parmesan, parsley and garlic over fish, introduce in the oven again and cook for 5 minutes more.
3. Divide between plates and serve.
Enjoy!

Nutrition: calories 240, fat 12, fiber 1, carbs 0.6, protein 25

Sour Cream Salmon

Preparation time: 10 minutes
Cooking time: 15 minutes
Servings: 4

Ingredients:
4 salmon fillets
A drizzle of olive oil
Salt and black pepper to the taste
1/3 cup parmesan, grated
1 and ½ teaspoon mustard
½ cup sour cream

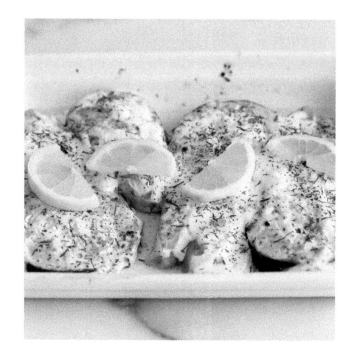

Directions:
1. Place salmon on a lined baking sheet, season with salt and pepper and drizzle the oil.
2. In a bowl, mix sour cream with parmesan, mustard, salt and pepper and stir well.
3. Spoon this sour cream mix over salmon, introduce in the oven at 350 degrees F and bake for 15 minutes.
4. Divide between plates and serve.
Enjoy!

Nutrition: calories 200, fat 6, fiber 1, carbs 4, protein 20

Grilled Salmon

Preparation time: 30 minutes
Cooking time: 10 minutes
Servings: 4

Ingredients:
4 salmon fillets
1 tablespoon olive oil
Salt and black pepper to the taste
1 teaspoon cumin, ground
1 teaspoon sweet paprika
½ teaspoon ancho chili powder
1 teaspoon onion powder
For the salsa:
1 small red onion, chopped
1 avocado, pitted, peeled and chopped
2 tablespoons cilantro, chopped
Juice from 2 limes
Salt and black pepper to the taste

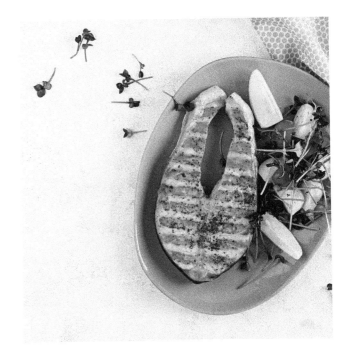

Directions:
1. In a bowl, mix salt, pepper, chili powder, onion powder, paprika and cumin.
2. Rub salmon with this mix, drizzle the oil and rub again and cook on preheated grill for 4 minutes on each side.
3. Meanwhile, in a bowl, mix avocado with red onion, salt, pepper, cilantro and lime juice and stir.
4. Divide salmon between plates and top each fillet with avocado salsa.
Enjoy!

Nutrition: calories 300, fat 14, fiber 4, carbs 5, protein 20

Tasty Tuna Cakes

Preparation time: 10 minutes
Cooking time: 10 minutes
Servings: 12

Ingredients:
15 ounces canned tuna, drain well and flaked
3 eggs
½ teaspoon dill, dried
1 teaspoon parsley, dried
½ cup red onion, chopped
1 teaspoon garlic powder
Salt and black pepper to the taste
Oil for frying

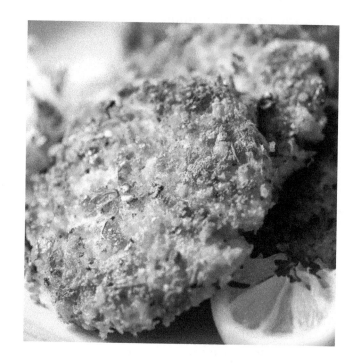

Directions:
1. In a bowl, mix tuna with salt, pepper, dill, parsley, onion, garlic powder and eggs and stir well.
2. Shape your cakes and place on a plate.
3. Heat up a pan with some oil over medium high heat, add tuna cakes, cook for 5 minutes on each side.
4. Divide between plates and serve.
Enjoy!

Nutrition: calories 140, fat 2, fiber 1, carbs 0.6, protein 6

Very Tasty Cod

Preparation time: 10 minutes
Cooking time: 20 minutes
Servings: 4

Ingredients:
1 pound cod, cut into medium pieces
Salt and black pepper to the taste
2 green onions, chopped
3 garlic cloves, minced
3 tablespoons soy sauce
1 cup fish stock
1 tablespoons balsamic vinegar
1 tablespoon ginger, grated
½ teaspoon chili pepper, crushed

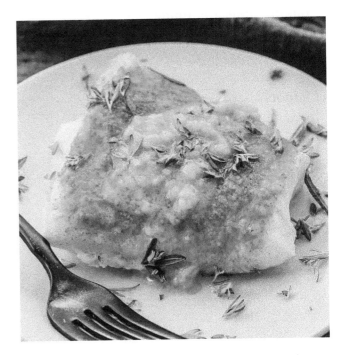

Directions:
1. Heat up a pan over medium high heat, add fish pieces and brown it a few minutes on each side.
2. Add garlic, green onions, salt, pepper, soy sauce, fish stock, vinegar, chili pepper and ginger, stir, cover, reduce heat and cook for 20 minutes.
3. Divide between plates and serve.
Enjoy!

Nutrition: calories 154, fat 3, fiber 0.5, carbs 4, protein 24

Tasty Sea Bass With Capers

Preparation time: 10 minutes
Cooking time: 15 minutes
Servings: 4

Ingredients:
1 lemon, sliced
1 pound sea bass fillet
2 tablespoons capers
2 tablespoons dill
Salt and black pepper to the taste

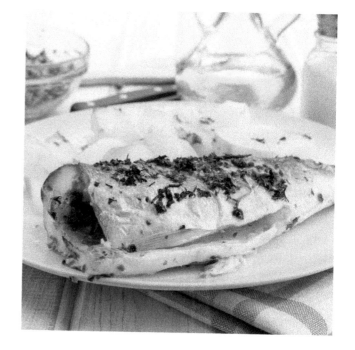

Directions:
1. Put sea bass fillet into a baking dish, season with salt and pepper, add capers, dill and lemon slices on top.
2. Introduce in the oven at 350 degrees F and bake for 15 minutes.
3. Divide between plates and serve.
Enjoy!

Nutrition: calories 150, fat 3, fiber 2, carbs 0.7, protein 5

Cod With Arugula

Preparation time: 10 minutes
Cooking time: 20 minutes
Servings: 2

Ingredients:
2 cod fillets
1 tablespoon olive oil
Salt and black pepper to the taste
Juice of 1 lemon
3 cup arugula
½ cup black olives, pitted and sliced
2 tablespoons capers
1 garlic clove, chopped

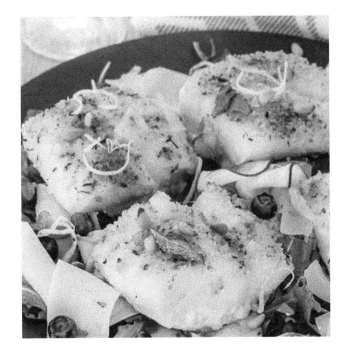

Directions:
1. Arrange fish fillets in a heatproof dish, season with salt, pepper, drizzle the oil and lemon juice, toss to coat, introduce in the oven at 450 degrees F and bake for 20 minutes.
2. In your food processor, mix arugula with salt, pepper, capers, olives and garlic and blend a bit.
3. Arrange fish on plates, top with arugula tapenade and serve.
Enjoy!

Nutrition: calories 240, fat 5, fiber 3, carbs 3, protein 10

Baked Halibut And Veggies

Preparation time: 10 minutes
Cooking time: 35 minutes
Servings: 2

Ingredients:
1 red bell pepper, roughly chopped
1 yellow bell pepper, roughly chopped
1 teaspoon balsamic vinegar
1 tablespoon olive oil
2 halibut fillets
2 cups baby spinach
Salt and black pepper to the taste
1 teaspoon cumin

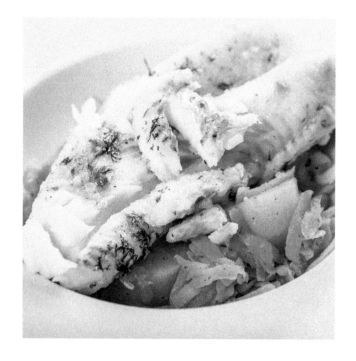

Directions:
1. In a bowl, mix bell peppers with salt, pepper, half of the oil and the vinegar, toss to coat well and transfer to a baking dish.
2. Introduce in the oven at 400 degrees F and bake for 20 minutes.
3. Heat up a pan with the rest of the oil over medium heat, add
fish, season with salt, pepper and cumin and brown on all sides.
4. Take the baking dish out of the oven, add spinach, stir gently and divide the whole mix between plates.
5. Add fish on the side, sprinkle some more salt and pepper and serve.
Enjoy!

Nutrition: calories 230, fat 12, fiber 1, carbs 4, protein 9

Tasty Fish Curry

Preparation time: 10 minutes
Cooking time: 25 minutes
Servings: 4

Ingredients:
4 white fish fillets
½ teaspoon mustard seeds
Salt and black pepper to the taste
2 green chilies, chopped
1 teaspoon ginger, grated
1 teaspoon curry powder
¼ teaspoon cumin, ground
4 tablespoons coconut oil
1 small red onion, chopped
1 inch turmeric root, grated
¼ cup cilantro
1 and ½ cups coconut cream
3 garlic cloves, minced

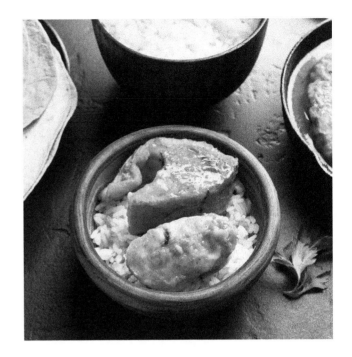

Directions:
1. Heat up a pot with half of the coconut oil over medium heat, add mustard seeds and cook for 2 minutes.
2. Add ginger, onion and garlic, stir and cook for 5 minutes.
3. Add turmeric, curry powder, chilies and cumin, stir and cook for 5 minutes more.
4. Add coconut milk, salt and pepper, stir, bring to a boil and cook for 15 minutes.
5. Heat up another pan with the rest of the oil over medium heat, add fish, stir and cook for 3 minutes.
6. Add this to the curry sauce, stir and cook for 5 minutes more.
7. Add cilantro, stir, divide into bowls and serve.
Enjoy!

Nutrition: calories 500, fat 34, fiber 7, carbs 6, protein 44

Delicious Shrimp

Preparation time: *10 minutes*
Cooking time: 10 minutes
Servings: 4

Ingredients:
2 tablespoons olive oil
1 tablespoon ghee
1 pound shrimp, peeled and deveined
2 tablespoons lemon juice
2 tablespoons garlic, minced
1 tablespoon lemon zest
Salt and black pepper to the taste

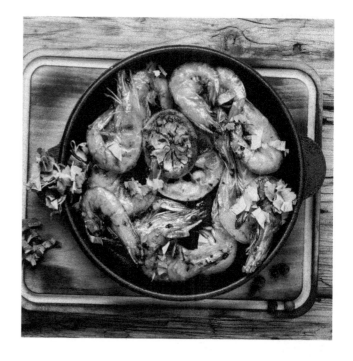

Directions:
1. Heat up a pan with the oil and the ghee over medium high heat, add shrimp and cook for 2 minutes.
2. Add garlic, stir and cook for 4 minutes more.
3. Add lemon juice, lemon zest, salt and pepper, stir, take off heat and serve.
Enjoy!

Nutrition: calories 149, fat 1, fiber 3, carbs 1, protein 6

Roasted Barramundi

Preparation time: 10 minutes
Cooking time: 12 minutes
Servings: 4

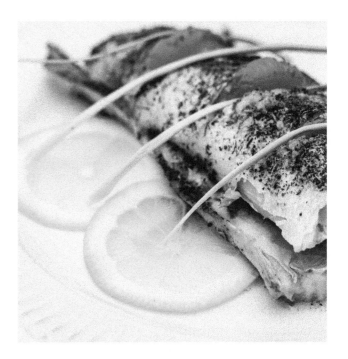

Ingredients:
2 barramundi fillets
2 teaspoon olive oil
2 teaspoons Italian seasoning
¼ cup green olives, pitted and chopped
¼ cup cherry tomatoes, chopped
¼ cup black olives, chopped
1 tablespoon lemon zest
2 tablespoons lemon zest
Salt and black pepper to the taste
2 tablespoons parsley, chopped
1 tablespoon olive oil

Directions:
1. Rub fish with salt, pepper, Italian seasoning and 2 teaspoons olive oil, transfer to a baking dish and leave aside for now.
2. Meanwhile, in a bowl, mix tomatoes with all the olives, salt, pepper, lemon zest and lemon juice, parsley and 1 tablespoon olive oil and toss everything well.
3. Introduce fish in the oven at 400 degrees F and bake for 12 minutes.
4. Divide fish on plates, top with tomato relish and serve.
Enjoy!

Nutrition: calories 150, fat 4, fiber 2, carbs 1, protein 10

Coconut Shrimp

Preparation time: 10 minutes
Cooking time: 13 minutes
Servings: 4

Ingredients:
1 pound shrimp, peeled and deveined
Salt and black pepper to the taste
4 cherry tomatoes, chopped
2 cups sugar snap peas, sliced lengthwise
1 red bell pepper, sliced
1 tablespoon olive oil
½ cup cilantro, chopped
1 tablespoon garlic, minced
½ cup green onion, chopped
½ teaspoon red pepper flakes
10 ounces coconut milk
2 tablespoons lime juice

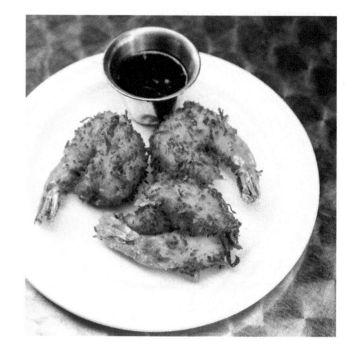

Directions:
1. Heat up a pan with the oil over medium high heat, add snap peas and stir-fry for 2 minutes.
2. Add pepper and cook for 3 minutes more.
3. Add cilantro, garlic, green onions and pepper flakes, stir and cook for 1 minute.
4. Add tomatoes and coconut milk, stir and simmer everything for 5 minutes.
5. Add shrimp and lime juice, stir and cook for 3 minutes.
6. Season with salt and pepper, stir and serve hot.
Enjoy!

Nutrition: calories 150, fat 3, fiber 3, carbs 1, protein 7

Shrimp And Noodle Salad

Preparation time: 10 minutes
Cooking time: 0 minutes
Servings: 4

Ingredients:
1 cucumber, cut with a spiralizer
½ cup basil, chopped
½ pound shrimp, already cooked, peeled and devei
Salt and black pepper to the taste
1 tablespoon stevia
2 teaspoons fish sauce
2 tablespoons lime juice
2 teaspoons chili garlic sauce

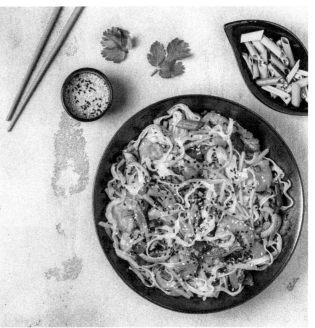

Directions:
1. Put cucumber noodles on a paper towel, cover with another one and press well.
2. Put into a bowl and mix with basil, shrimp, salt and pepper.
3. In another bowl, mix stevia with fish sauce, lime juice and chili sauce and whisk well.
4. Add this to shrimp salad, toss to coat well and serve.
Enjoy!

Nutrition: calories 130, fat 2, fiber 3, carbs 1, protein 6

Roasted Mahi Mahi And Salsa

Preparation time: 10 minutes
Cooking time: 16 minutes
Servings: 2

Ingredients:
2 mahi-mahi fillets
½ cup yellow onion, chopped
4 teaspoons olive oil
1 teaspoon Greek seasoning
1 teaspoon garlic, minced
1 green bell pepper, chopped
½ cup canned tomato salsa
2 tablespoons kalamata olives,
pitted and chopped
¼ cup chicken stock
Salt and black pepper to the taste
2 tablespoons feta cheese, crumbled

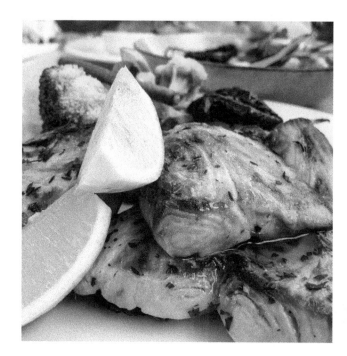

Directions:
1. Heat up a pan with 2 teaspoons oil over medium heat, add bell pepper and onion, stir and cook for 3 minutes.
2. Add Greek seasoning and garlic, stir and cook for 1 minute more.
3. Add stock, olives and salsa, stir again and cook until the mixture thickens for 5 minutes.
4. Transfer to a bowl and leave aside for now.
5. Heat up the pan again with the rest of the oil over medium heat, add fish, season with salt and pepper and cook for 2 minutes.
6. Flip, cook for 2 minutes more and transfer to a baking dish.
7. Spoon salsa over fish, introduce in the oven and bake at 425 degrees F for 6 minutes.
8. Sprinkle feta on top and serve hot.
Enjoy!

Nutrition: calories 200, fat 5, fiber 2, carbs 2, protein 7

Spicy Shrimp

Preparation time: 10 minutes
Cooking time: 8 minutes
Servings: 2

Ingredients:
½ pound big shrimp, peeled and deveined
2 teaspoons Worcestershire sauce
2 teaspoons olive oil
Juice of 1 lemon
Salt and black pepper to the taste
1 teaspoon Creole seasoning

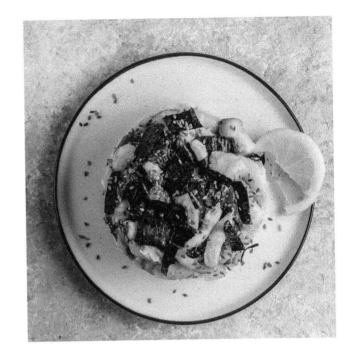

Directions:
1. Arrange shrimp in one layer in a baking dish, season with salt and pepper and drizzle the oil.
2. Add Worcestershire sauce, lemon juice and sprinkle Creole seasoning.
3. Toss shrimp a bit, introduce in the oven, set it on the broiler and cook for 8 minutes.
4. Divide between 2 plates and serve.
Enjoy!

Nutrition: calories 120, fat 3, fiber 1, carbs 2, protein 6

Shrimp Stew

Preparation time: 10 minutes
Cooking time: 15 minutes
Servings: 6

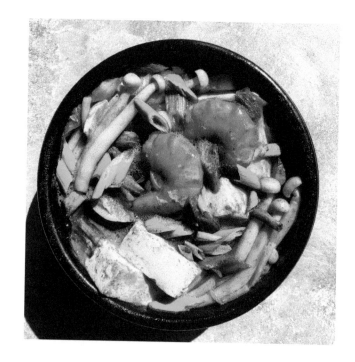

Ingredients:
¼ cup yellow onion, chopped
¼ cup olive oil
1 garlic clove, minced
1 and ½ pounds shrimp, peeled and deveined
¼ cup red pepper, roasted and chopped
14 ounces canned tomatoes, chopped
¼ cup cilantro, chopped
2 tablespoons sriracha sauce
1 cup coconut milk
Salt and black pepper to the taste
2 tablespoons lime juice

Directions:
1. Heat up a pan with the oil over medium heat, add onion, stir and cook for 4 minutes.
2. Add peppers and garlic, stir and cook for 4 minutes more.
3. Add cilantro, tomatoes and shrimp, stir and cook until shrimp turn pink.
4. Add coconut milk and sriracha sauce, stir and bring to a gentle simmer.
5. Add salt, pepper and lime juice, stir, transfer to bowls and serve.
Enjoy!

Nutrition: calories 250, fat 12, fiber 3, carbs 5, protein 20

Shrimp Alfredo

Preparation time: 10 minutes
Cooking time: 20 minutes
Servings: 4

Ingredients:
8 ounces mushrooms, chopped
1 asparagus bunch, cut into medium pieces
1 pound shrimp, peeled and deveined
Salt and black pepper to the taste
1 spaghetti squash, cut in halves
2 tablespoons olive oil
2 teaspoons Italian seasoning
1 yellow onion, chopped
1 teaspoon red pepper flakes, crushed
¼ cup ghee
1 cup parmesan cheese, grated
2 garlic cloves, minced
1 cup heavy cream

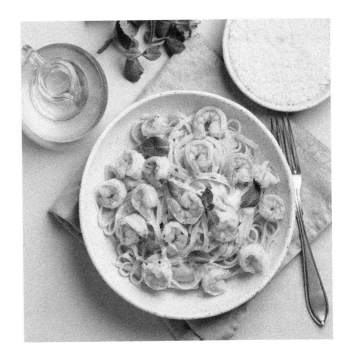

Directions:
1. Place squash halves on a lined baking sheet, introduce in the oven at 425 degrees F and roast for 40 minutes.
2. Scoop insides and put into a bowl.
3. Put water in a pot, add some salt, bring to a boil over medium heat, add asparagus, steam for a couple of minutes, transfer to a bowl filled with ice water, drain and leave aside as well.
4. Heat up a pan with the oil over medium heat, add onions and mushrooms, stir and cook for 7 minutes.
5. Add pepper flakes, Italian seasoning, salt, pepper, squash and asparagus, stir and cook for a few minutes more.
6. Heat up another pan with the ghee over medium heat, add heavy cream, garlic and parmesan, stir and cook for 5 minutes.
7. Add shrimp to this pan, stir and cook for 7 minutes.
8. Divide veggies on plates, top with shrimp and sauce and serve.
Enjoy!

Nutrition: calories 455, fat 6, fiber 5, carbs 4, protein 13

Shrimp And Snow Peas Soup

Preparation time: 10 minutes
Cooking time: 10 minutes
Servings: 4

Ingredients:
4 scallions, chopped
1 and ½ tablespoons coconut oil
1 small ginger root, finely chopped
8 cups chicken stock
¼ cup coconut aminos
5 ounces canned bamboo shoots, sliced
Black pepper to the taste
¼ teaspoon fish sauce
1 pound shrimp, peeled and deveined
½ pound snow peas
1 tablespoon sesame oil
½ tablespoon chili oil

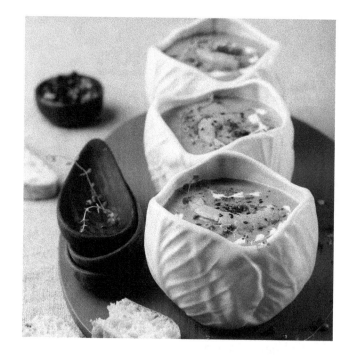

Directions:
1. Heat up a pot with the coconut oil over medium heat, add scallions and ginger, stir and cook for 2 minutes.
2. Add coconut aminos, stock, black pepper and fish sauce, stir and bring to a boil.
3. Add shrimp, snow peas and bamboo shoots, stir and cook for 3 minutes.
4. Add sesame oil and hot chili oil, stir, divide into bowls and serve.
Enjoy!

Nutrition: calories 200, fat 3, fiber 2, carbs 4, protein 14

Simple Mussels Dish

Preparation time: 5 minutes
Cooking time: 5 minutes
Servings: 4

Ingredients:
2 pound mussels, debearded and scrubbed
2 garlic cloves, minced
1 tablespoon ghee
A splash of lemon juice

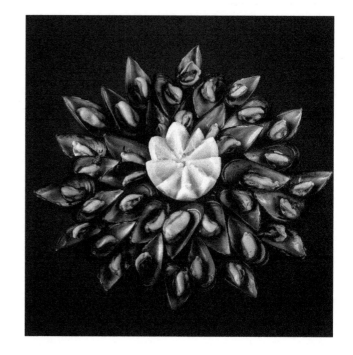

Directions:
1. Put some water in a pot, add mussels, bring to a boil over medium heat, cook for 5 minutes, take off heat, discard unopened mussels and transfer them to a bowl.
2. In another bowl, mix ghee with garlic and lemon juice, whisk and heat up in the microwave for 1 minute.
3. Pour over mussels and serve them right away.
Enjoy!

Nutrition: calories 50, fat 1, fiber 0, carbs 0.5, protein 2

Simple Fried Calamari And Tasty Sauce

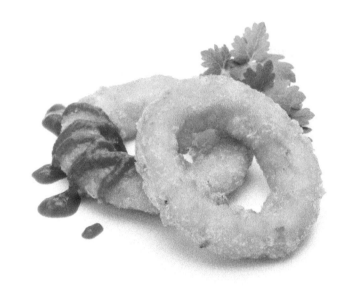

Preparation time: 10 minutes
Cooking time: 20 minutes
Servings: 2

Ingredients:
1 squid, cut into medium rings
A pinch of cayenne pepper
1 egg, whisked
2 tablespoons coconut flour
Salt and black pepper to the taste
Coconut oil for frying
1 tablespoons lemon juice
4 tablespoons mayo
1 teaspoon sriracha sauce

Directions:
1. Season squid rings with salt, pepper and cayenne and put them in a bowl.
2. In a bowl, whisk the egg with salt, pepper and coconut flour and whisk well.
3. Dredge calamari rings in this mix.
4. Heat up a pan with enough coconut oil over medium heat, add calamari rings, cook them until they become gold on both
sides.
5. Transfer to paper towels, drain grease and put in a bowl.
6. In another bowl, mix mayo with lemon juice and sriracha sauce, stir well and serve your calamari rings with this sauce on the side.
Enjoy!

Nutrition: calories 345, fat 32, fiber 3, carbs 3, protein 13

Baked Calamari And Shrimp

Preparation time: 10 minutes
Cooking time: 20 minutes
Servings: 1

Ingredients:
8 ounces calamari, cut into medium rings
7 ounces shrimp, peeled and deveined
1 eggs
3 tablespoons coconut flour
1 tablespoon coconut oil
2 tablespoons avocado, chopped
1 teaspoon tomato paste
1 tablespoon mayonnaise
A splash of Worcestershire sauce
1 teaspoon lemon juice
2 lemon slices
Salt and black pepper to the taste
½ teaspoon turmeric

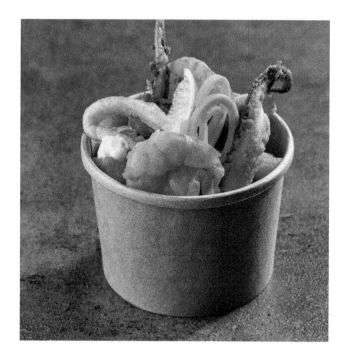

Directions:
1. In a bowl, whisk the egg with coconut oil.
2. Add calamari rings and shrimp and toss to coat.
3. In another bowl, mix flour with salt, pepper and turmeric and stir.
4. Dredge calamari and shrimp in this mix, place everything on a lined baking sheet, introduce in the oven at 400 degrees F and bake for 10 minutes.
5. Flip calamari and shrimp and bake for 10 minutes more.
6. Meanwhile, in a bowl, mix avocado with mayo and tomato paste and mash using a fork.
7. Add Worcestershire sauce, lemon juice, salt and pepper and stir well.
8. Divide baked calamari and shrimp on plates and serve with the sauce and lemon juice on the side.
Enjoy!

Nutrition: calories 368, fat 23, fiber 3, carbs 10, protein 34

Octopus Salad

Preparation time: 10 minutes
Cooking time: 40 minutes
Servings: 2

Ingredients:
21 ounces octopus, rinsed
Juice of 1 lemon
4 celery stalks, chopped
3 ounces olive oil
Salt and black pepper to the taste
4 tablespoons parsley, chopped

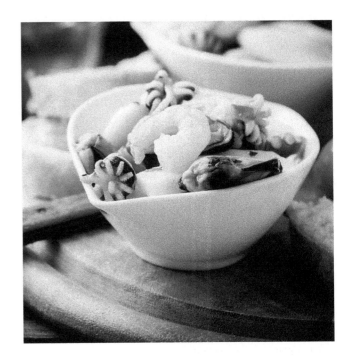

Directions:
1. Put the octopus in a pot, add water to cover, cover pot, bring to a boil over medium heat, cook for 40 minutes, drain and leave aside to cool down.
2. Chop octopus and put it in a salad bowl.
3. Add celery stalks, parsley, oil and lemon juice and toss well.
4. Season with salt and pepper, toss again and serve.
Enjoy!

Nutrition: calories 140, fat 10, fiber 3, carbs 6, protein 23

Clam Chowder

Preparation time: 10 minutes
Cooking time: 2 hours
Servings: 4

Ingredients:
1 cup celery stalks, chopped
Salt and black pepper to the taste
1 teaspoon thyme, ground
2 cups chicken stock
14 ounces canned baby clams
2 cups whipping cream
1 cup onion, chopped
13 bacon slices, chopped

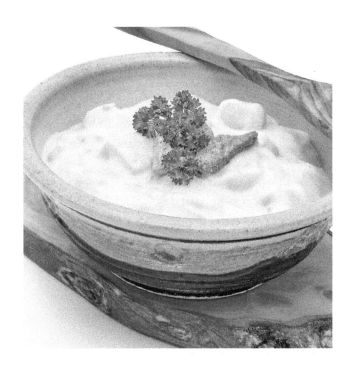

Directions:
1. Heat up a pan over medium heat, add bacon slices, brown them and transfer to a bowl.
2. Heat up the same pan over medium heat, add celery and onion, stir and cook for 5 minutes.
3. Transfer everything to your Crockpot, also add bacon, baby clams, salt, pepper, stock, thyme and whipping cream, stir and cook on High for 2 hours.
4. Divide into bowls and serve.
Enjoy!

Nutrition: calories 420, fat 22, fiber 0, carbs 5, protein 25

Delicious Flounder And Shrimp

Preparation time: 10 minutes
Cooking time: 20 minutes
Servings: 4

Ingredients:

For the seasoning:

2 teaspoons onion powder, 2 teaspoons thyme, dried
2 teaspoons sweet paprika, 2 teaspoons garlic powder
Salt and black pepper to the taste
½ teaspoon allspice, ground
1 teaspoon oregano, dried
A pinch of cayenne pepper
¼ teaspoon nutmeg, ground
¼ teaspoon cloves
A pinch of cinnamon powder
For the etouffee:, 2 shallots, chopped
1 tablespoon ghee, 8 ounces bacon, sliced
1 green bell pepper, chopped
1 celery stick, chopped
2 tablespoons coconut flour, 1 tomato, chopped

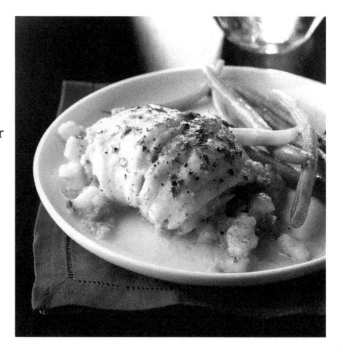

4 garlic cloves, minced, 8 ounces shrimp, peeled, deveined and chopped, 2 cups chicken stock, 1 tablespoon coconut milk A handful parsley, chopped, 1 teaspoon Tabasco sauce, Salt and black pepper to the taste. For the flounder:, 4 flounder fillets, 2 tablespoons ghee

Directions:

1. In a bowl, mix paprika with thyme, garlic and onion powder, salt, pepper, oregano, allspice, cayenne pepper, cloves, nutmeg and cinnamon and stir.
2. Reserve 2 tablespoons of this mix, rub the flounder with the rest and leave aside.
3. Heat up a pan over medium heat, add bacon, stir and cook for 6 minutes.
4. Add celery, bell pepper, shallots and 1 tablespoon ghee, stir and cook for 4 minutes.
5. Add tomato and garlic, stir and cook for 4 minutes.
6. Add coconut flour and reserved seasoning, stir and cook for 2 minutes more.
7. Add chicken stock and bring to a simmer.
8. Meanwhile, heat up a pan with 2 tablespoons ghee over medium high heat, add fish, cook for 2 minutes, flip and cut for 2 minutes more. Add shrimp to the pan with the stock, stir and cook for 2 minutes.
9. Add parsley, salt, pepper, coconut milk and Tabasco sauce, stir and take off heat.
10. Divide fish on plates, top with the shrimp sauce and serve.
Enjoy!

Nutrition: calories 200, fat 5, fiber 7, carbs 4, protein 20

Shrimp Salad

Preparation time: 10 minutes
Cooking time: 10 minutes
*Serving*s: 4

Ingredients:
2 tablespoons olive oil
1 pound shrimp, peeled and deveined
Salt and black pepper to the taste
2 tablespoons lime juice
3 endives, leaves separated
3 tablespoons parsley, chopped
2 teaspoons mint, chopped
1 tablespoon tarragon, chopped
1 tablespoon lemon juice
2 tablespoons mayonnaise
1 teaspoon lime zest
½ cup sour cream

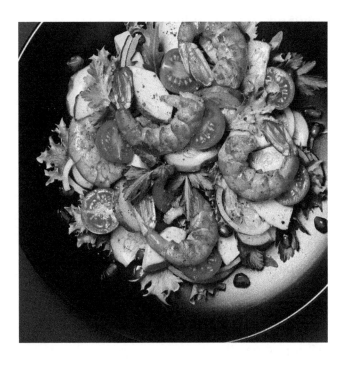

Directions:
1. In a bowl, mix shrimp with salt, pepper and the olive oil, toss to coat and spread them on a lined baking sheet.
2. Introduce shrimp in the oven at 400 degrees F and bake for 10 minutes.
3. Add lime juice, toss them to coat again and leave aside for now.
4. In a bowl, mix mayo with sour cream, lime zest, lemon juice, salt, pepper, tarragon, mint and parsley and stir very well.
5. Chop shrimp, add to salad dressing, toss to coat everything and spoon into endive leaves.
6. Serve right away.
Enjoy!

Nutrition: calories 200, fat 11, fiber 2, carbs 1, protein 13

Delicious Oysters

Preparation time: 10 minutes
Cooking time: 0 minutes
Servings: 4

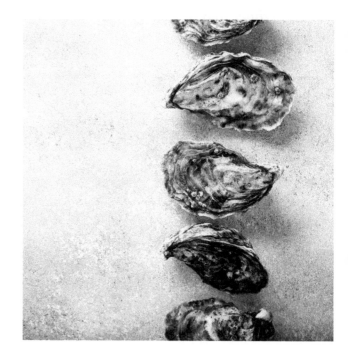

Ingredients:
12 oysters, shucked
Juice of 1 lemon
Juice from 1 orange
Zest from 1 orange
Juice from 1 lime
Zest from 1 lime
2 tablespoons ketchup
1 Serrano chili pepper, chopped
1 cup tomato juice
½ teaspoon ginger, grated
¼ teaspoon garlic, minced
Salt to the taste
¼ cup olive oil
¼ cup cilantro, chopped
¼ cup scallions, chopped

Directions:
1. In a bowl, mix lemon juice, orange juice, orange zest, lime juice and zest, ketchup, chili pepper, tomato juice, ginger, garlic, oil, scallions, cilantro and salt and stir well.
2. Spoon this into oysters and serve them.
Enjoy!

Nutrition: calories 100, fat 1, fiber 0, carbs 2, protein 5

Incredible Salmon Rolls

Preparation time: 10 minutes
Cooking time: 0 minutes
Servings: 12

Ingredients:
2 nori seeds
1 small avocado, pitted, peeled
and finely chopped
6 ounces smoked salmon. Sliced
4 ounces cream cheese
1 cucumber, sliced
1 teaspoon wasabi paste
Picked ginger for serving

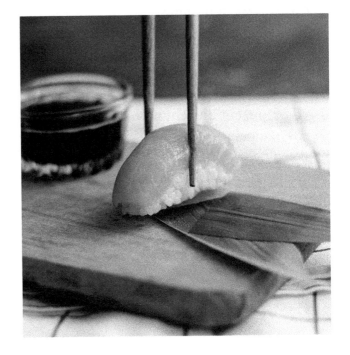

Directions:
1. Place nori sheets on a sushi mat.
2. Divide salmon slices on them and also avocado and cucumber slices.
3. In a bowl, mix cream cheese with wasabi paste and stir well.
4. Spread this over cucumber slices, roll your nori sheets, press well, cut each into 6 pieces and serve with pickled ginger.
Enjoy!

Nutrition: calories 80, fat 6, fiber 1, carbs 2, protein 4

Salmon Skewers

Preparation time: 10 minutes
Cooking time: 8 minutes
Servings: 4

Ingredients:
12 ounces salmon fillet, cubed
1 red onion, cut into chunks
½ red bell pepper cut in chunks
½ green bell pepper cut in chunks
½ orange bell pepper cut in chunks
Juice from 1 lemon
Salt and black pepper to the taste
A drizzle of olive oil

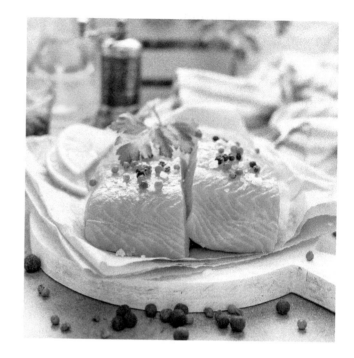

Directions:
1. Thread skewers with onion, red, green and orange pepper and salmon cubes.
2. Season them with salt and pepper, drizzle oil and lemon juice and place them on preheated grill over medium high heat.
3. Cook for 4 minutes on each side, divide between plates and serve.
Enjoy!

Nutrition: calories 150, fat 3, fiber 6, carbs 3, protein 8

Grilled Shrimp

Preparation time: 20 minutes
Cooking time: 10 minutes
Servings: 4

Ingredients:
1 pound shrimp, peeled and deveined
1 tablespoon lemon juice
1 garlic clove, minced
½ cup basil leaves
1 tablespoon pine nuts, toasted
2 tablespoons parmesan, grated
2 tablespoons olive oil
Salt and black pepper to the taste

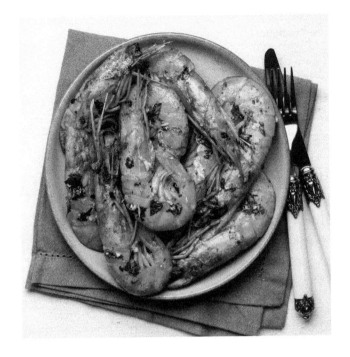

Directions:
1. In your food processor, mix parmesan with basil, garlic, pine nuts, oil, salt, pepper and lemon juice and blend well.
2. Transfer this to a bowl, add shrimp, toss to coat and leave aside for 20 minutes.
3. Thread skewers with marinated shrimp, place them on preheated grill over medium high heat, cook for 3 minutes, flip and cook for 3 more minutes.
4. Arrange on plates and serve.
Enjoy!

Nutrition: calories 185, fat 11, fiber 0, carbs 2, protein 13

Calamari Salad

Preparation time: 30 minutes
Cooking time: 4 minutes
Servings: 4

Ingredients:
2 long red chilies, chopped
2 small red chilies, chopped
2 garlic cloves, minced
3 green onions, chopped
1 tablespoon balsamic vinegar
Salt and black pepper to the taste
Juice of 1 lemon
6 pounds calamari hoods, tentacles reserved
3.5 ounces olive oil
3 ounces rocket for serving

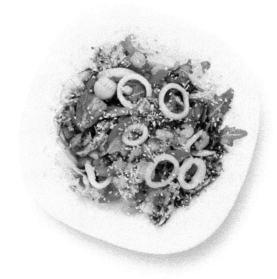

Directions:
1. In a bowl, mix long red chilies with small red chilies, green onions, vinegar, half of the oil, garlic, salt, pepper and lemon juice and stir well.
2. Place calamari and tentacles in a bowl, season with salt and pepper, drizzle the rest of the oil, toss to coat and place on preheated grill over medium high heat.
3. Cook for 2 minutes on each side and transfer to the chili marinade you've made.
4. Toss to coat and leave aside for 30 minutes.
5. Arrange rocket on plates, top with calamari and its marinade and serve.
Enjoy!

Nutrition: calories 200, fat 4, fiber 2, carbs 2, protein 7

Cod Salad

Preparation time: 2 hours and 10 minutes
Cooking time: 20 minutes
Servings: 8

Ingredients:
2 cups jarred pimiento peppers, chopped
2 pounds salt cod
1 cup parsley, chopped
1 cup kalamata olives, pitted and chopped
6 tablespoons capers
¾ cup olive oil
Salt and black pepper to the taste
Juice from 2 lemons
4 garlic cloves, minced
2 celery ribs, chopped
½ teaspoon red chili flakes
1 escarole head, leaves separated

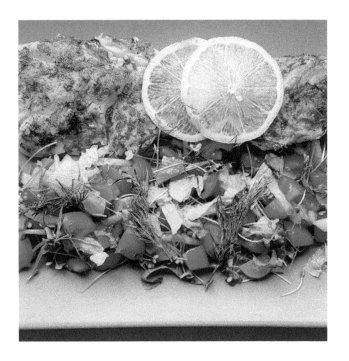

Directions:
1. Put cod in a pot, add water to cover, bring to a boil over medium heat, boil for 20 minutes, drain and cut into medium chunks.
2. Put cod in a salad bowl, add peppers, parsley, olives, capers, celery, garlic, lemon juice, salt, pepper, olive oil and chili
flakes and toss to coat.
3. Arrange escarole leaves on a platter, add cod salad and serve.
Enjoy!

Nutrition: calories 240, fat 4, fiber 2, carbs 6, protein 9

Sardines Salad

Preparation time: 10 minutes
Cooking time: 0 minutes
Servings: 1

Ingredients:
5 ounces canned sardines in oil
1 tablespoons lemon juice
1 small cucumber, chopped
½ tablespoon mustard
Salt and black pepper to the taste

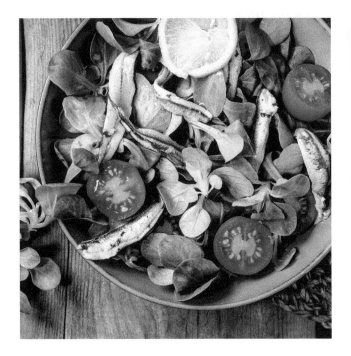

Directions:
1. Drain sardines, put them in a bowl and mash using a fork.
2. Add salt, pepper, cucumber, lemon juice and mustard, stir well and serve cold.
Enjoy!

Nutrition: calories 200, fat 20, fiber 1, carbs 0, protein 20

Italian Clams Delight

Preparation time: 10 minutes
Cooking time: 10 minutes
Servings: 6

Ingredients:
½ cup ghee
36 clams, scrubbed
1 teaspoon red pepper flakes, crushed
1 teaspoon parsley, chopped
5 garlic cloves, minced
1 tablespoon oregano, dried
2 cups white wine

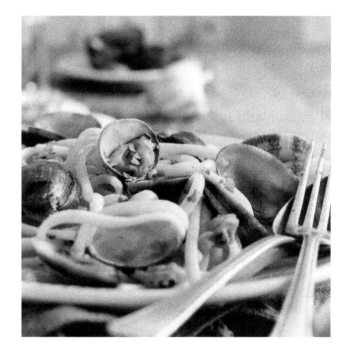

Directions:
1. Heat up a pan with the ghee over medium heat, add garlic, stir and cook for 1 minute.
2. Add parsley, oregano, wine and pepper flakes and stir well.
3. Add clams, stir, cover and cook for 10 minutes.
4. Discard unopened clams, ladle clams and their mix into bowls and serve.
Enjoy!

Nutrition: calories 224, fat 15, fiber 2, carbs 3, protein 4

Orange Glazed Salmon

Preparation time: 10 minutes
Cooking time: 10 minutes
Servings: 2

Ingredients:
2 lemons, sliced
1 pound wild salmon, skinless and cubed
¼ cup balsamic vinegar
¼ cup red orange juice
1 teaspoon coconut oil
1/3 cup orange marmalade, no sugar added

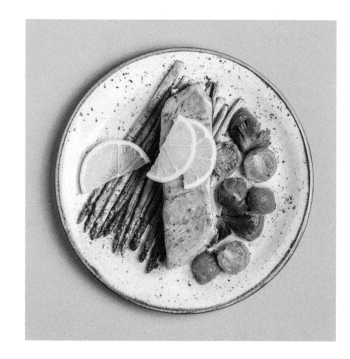

Directions:
1. Heat up a pot over medium heat, add vinegar, orange juice and marmalade, stir well, bring to a simmer for 1 minute, reduce temperature, cook until it thickens a bit and take off heat.
2. Arrange salmon and lemon slices on skewers and brush them on one side with the orange glaze.
3. Brush your kitchen grill with coconut oil and heat up over medium heat.
4. Place salmon kebabs on grill with glazed side down and cook for 4 minutes.
5. Flip kebabs, brush them with the rest of the orange glaze and cook for 4 minutes more.
6. Serve right away.
Enjoy!

Nutrition: calories 160, fat 3, fiber 2, carbs 1, protein 8

Delicious Tuna And Chimichurri Sauce

Preparation time: 10 minutes
Cooking time: 5 minutes
Servings: 4

Ingredients:
½ cup cilantro, chopped
1/3 cup olive oil
2 tablespoons olive oil
1 small red onion, chopped
3 tablespoon balsamic vinegar
2 tablespoons parsley, chopped
2 tablespoons basil, chopped
1 jalapeno pepper, chopped
1 pound sushi grade tuna steak
Salt and black pepper to the taste
1 teaspoon red pepper flakes
1 teaspoon thyme, chopped
A pinch of cayenne pepper
3 garlic cloves, minced
2 avocados, pitted, peeled and sliced
6 ounces baby arugula

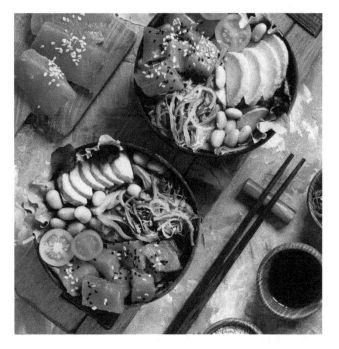

Directions:
1. In a bowl, mix 1/3 cup oil with jalapeno, vinegar, onion, cilantro, basil, garlic, parsley, pepper flakes, thyme, cayenne, salt and pepper, whisk well and leave aside for now.
2. Heat up a pan with the rest of the oil over medium high heat, add tuna, season with salt and pepper, cook for 2 minutes on each side, transfer to a cutting board, leave aside to cool down a bit and slice.
3. Mix arugula with half of the chimichurri mix you've made and toss to coat.
4. Divide arugula on plates, top with tuna slices, drizzle the rest of the chimichurri sauce and serve with avocado slices on the side.
Enjoy!

Nutrition: calories 186, fat 3, fiber 1, carbs 4, protein 20

Salmon Bites And Chili Sauce

Preparation time: 10 minutes
Cooking time: 15 minutes
Servings: 6

Ingredients:
1 and ¼ cups coconut, desiccated and unsweetened
1 pound salmon, cubed
1 egg
Salt and black pepper
1 tablespoon water
1/3 cup coconut flour
3 tablespoons coconut oil
For the sauce:
¼ teaspoon agar agar
3 garlic cloves, chopped
¾ cup water
4 Thai red chilies, chopped
¼ cup balsamic vinegar
½ cup stevia
A pinch of salt

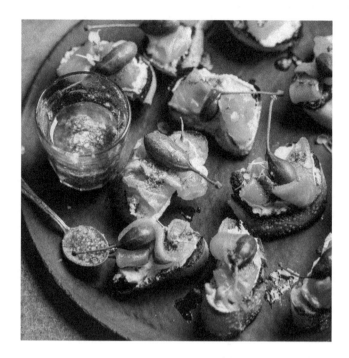

Directions:
1. In a bowl, mix flour with salt and pepper and stir.
2. In another bowl, whisk egg and 1 tablespoon water.
3. Put the coconut in a third bowl.
4. Dip salmon cubes in flour, egg and then in coconut and place them on a plate.
5. Heat up a pan with the coconut oil over medium high heat, add salmon bites, cook for 3 minutes on each side and transfer them to paper towels.
6. Heat up a pan with ¾ cup water over high heat, sprinkle agar agar and bring to a boil.
7. Cook for 3 minutes and take off heat.
8. In your blender, mix garlic with chilies, vinegar, stevia and a pinch of salt and blend well.
9. Transfer this to a small pan and heat up over medium high heat.
10. Stir, add agar mix and cook for 3 minutes.
11. Serve your salmon bites with chili sauce on the side.
Enjoy!

Nutrition: calories 50, fat 2, fiber 0, carbs 4, protein 2

Irish Clams

Preparation time: 10 minutes
Cooking time: 10 minutes
Servings: 4

Ingredients:
2 pounds clams, scrubbed
3 ounces pancetta
1 tablespoon olive oil
3 tablespoons ghee
2 garlic cloves, minced
1 bottle infused cider
Salt and black pepper to the taste
Juice of ½ lemon
1 small green apple, chopped
2 thyme springs, chopped

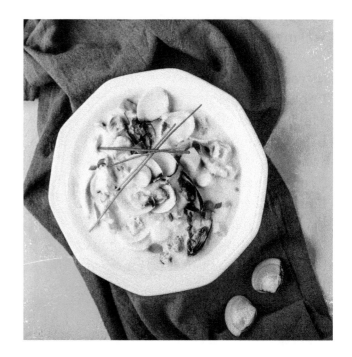

Directions:
1. Heat up a pan with the oil over medium high heat, add pancetta, brown for 3 minutes and reduce temperature to medium.
2. Add ghee, garlic, salt, pepper and shallot, stir and cook for 3 minutes.
3. Increase heat again, add cider, stir well and cook for 1 minute.
4. Add clams and thyme, cover pan and simmer for 5 minutes.
5. Discard unopened clams, add lemon juice and apple pieces, stir and divide into bowls.
6. Serve hot.
Enjoy!

Nutrition: calories 100, fat 2, fiber 1, carbs 1, protein 20

Seared Scallops And Roasted Grapes

Preparation time: 5 minutes
Cooking time: 10 minutes
Servings: 4

Ingredients:
1 pound scallops
3 tablespoons olive oil
1 shallot, chopped
3 garlic cloves, minced
2 cups spinach
1 cup chicken stock
1 romanesco lettuce head
1 and ½ cups red grapes, cut in halves
¼ cup walnuts, toasted and chopped
1 tablespoon ghee
Salt and black pepper to the taste

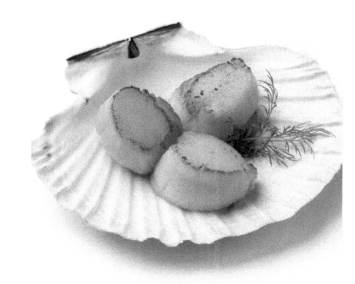

Directions:
1. Put romanesco in your food processor, blend and transfer to a bowl.
2. Heat up a pan with 2 tablespoons oil over medium high heat, add shallot and garlic, stir and cook for 1 minute.
3. Add romanesco, spinach and 1 cup stock, stir, cook for 3 minutes, blend using an immersion blender and take off heat.
4. Heat up another pan with 1 tablespoon oil and the ghee over medium high heat, add scallops, season with salt and pepper, cook for 2 minutes, flip and sear for 1 minute more.
5. Divide romanesco mix on plates, add scallops on the side, top with walnuts and grapes and serve.
Enjoy!

Nutrition: calories 300, fat 12, fiber 2, carbs 6, protein 20

Oysters And Pico De Gallo

Preparation time: 10 minutes
Cooking time: 10 minutes
Servings: 6

Ingredients:
18 oysters, scrubbed
A handful cilantro, chopped
2 tomatoes, chopped
1 jalapeno pepper, chopped
¼ cup red onion, finely chopped
Salt and black pepper to the taste
½ cup Monterey Jack cheese, shredded
2 limes, cut into wedges
Juice from 1 lime

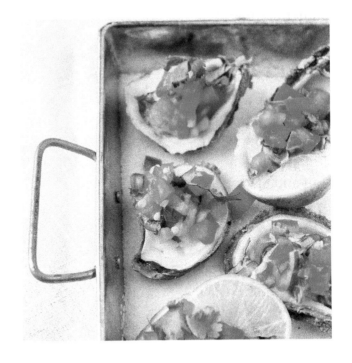

Directions:
1. In a bowl, mix onion with jalapeno, cilantro, tomatoes, salt, pepper and lime juice and stir well.
2. Place oysters on preheated grill over medium high heat, cover grill and cook for 7 minutes until they open.
3. Transfer opened oysters to a heatproof dish and discard unopened ones.
4. Top oysters with cheese and introduce in preheated broiler for 1 minute.
5. Arrange oysters on a platter, top each with tomatoes mix you've made earlier and serve with lime wedges on the side.
Enjoy!

Nutrition: calories 70, fat 2, fiber 0, carbs 1, protein 1

Grilled Squid And Tasty Guacamole

Preparation time: 10 minutes
Cooking time: 10 minutes
Servings: 2

Ingredients:
2 medium squids, tentacles separated
and tubes scored lengthwise
A drizzle of olive oil
Juice from 1 lime
Salt and black pepper to the taste
For the guacamole:
2 avocados, pitted, peeled and chopped
Some coriander springs, chopped
2 red chilies, chopped
1 tomato, chopped
1 red onion, chopped
Juice from 2 limes

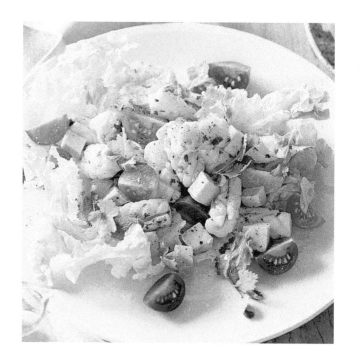

Directions:
1. Season squid and squid tentacles with salt, pepper, drizzle some olive oil and massage well.
2. Place on preheated grill over medium high heat score side down and cook for 2 minutes.
3. Flip and cook for 2 minutes more and transfer to a bowl.
4. Add juice from 1 lime, toss to coat and keep warm.
5. Put avocado in a bowl and mash using a fork.
6. Add coriander, chilies, tomato, onion and juice from 2 limes and stir well everything.
7. Divide squid on plates, top with guacamole and serve.
Enjoy!

Nutrition: calories 500, fat 43, fiber 6, carbs 7, protein 20

POULTRY

Delicious Chicken Nuggets

Preparation time: 10 minutes
Cooking time: 15 minutes
Servings: 2

Ingredients:
½ cup coconut flour
1 egg
2 tablespoons garlic powder
2 chicken breasts, cubed
Salt and black pepper to the taste
½ cup ghee

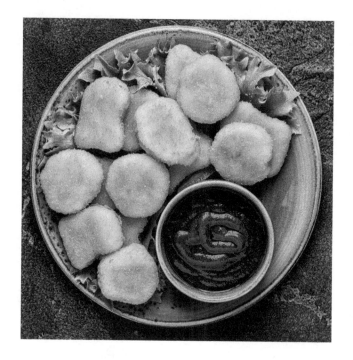

Directions:
1. In a bowl, mix garlic powder with coconut flour, salt and pepper and stir.
2. In another bowl, whisk egg well.
3. Dip chicken breast cubes in egg mix, then in flour mix.
4. Heat up a pan with the ghee over medium heat, drop chicken nuggets and cook them for 5 minutes on each side.
5. Transfer to paper towels, drain grease and then serve them with some tasty ketchup on the side.
Enjoy!

Nutrition: calories 60, fat 3, fiber 0.2, carbs 3, protein 4

Chicken Wings And Tasty Mint Chutney

Preparation time: 20 minutes
Cooking time: 25 minutes
Servings: 6

Ingredients:
18 chicken wings, cut in halves
1 tablespoon turmeric
1 tablespoon cumin, ground
1 tablespoon ginger, grated
1 tablespoon coriander, ground
1 tablespoon paprika
A pinch of cayenne pepper
Salt and black pepper to the taste
2 tablespoons olive oil
For the chutney:
Juice of ½ lime
1 cup mint leaves
1 small ginger piece, chopped
¾ cup cilantro
1 tablespoon olive oil
1 tablespoon water
Salt and black pepper to the taste
1 Serrano pepper

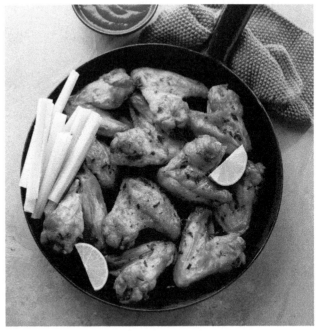

Directions:
1. In a bowl, mix 1 tablespoon ginger with cumin, coriander, paprika, turmeric, salt, pepper, cayenne and 2 tablespoons oil and stir well.
2. Add chicken wings pieces to this mix, toss to coat well and keep in the fridge for 20 minutes.
3. Heat up your grill over high heat, add marinated wings, cook for 25 minutes, turning them from time to time and transfer to a bowl.
4. In your blender, mix mint with cilantro, 1 small ginger pieces, juice from ½ lime, 1 tablespoon olive oil, salt, pepper, water and Serrano pepper and blend very well.
5. Serve your chicken wings with this sauce on the side.
Enjoy!

Nutrition: calories 100, fat 5, fiber 1, carbs 1, protein 9

Chicken Meatballs

Preparation time: 10 minutes
Cooking time: 15 minutes
Servings: 3

Ingredients:
1 pound chicken meat, ground
Salt and black pepper to the taste
2 tablespoons ranch dressing
½ cup almond flour
¼ cup cheddar cheese, grated
1 tablespoon dry ranch seasoning
¼ cup hot sauce+ some more for serving
1 egg

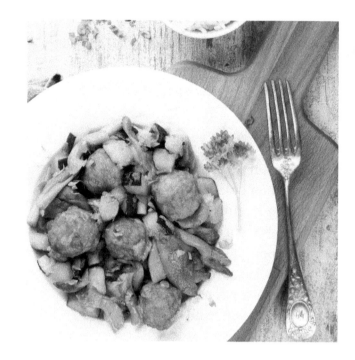

Directions:
1. In a bowl, mix chicken meat with salt, pepper, ranch dressing, flour, dry ranch seasoning, cheddar cheese, hot sauce and the egg and Stir very well.
2. Shape 9 meatballs, place them all on a lined baking sheet and bake at 500 degrees F for 15 minutes.
3. Serve chicken meatballs with hot sauce on the side.
Enjoy!

Nutrition: calories 156, fat 11, fiber 1, carbs 2, protein 12

Tasty Grilled Chicken Wings

Preparation time: 2 hours and 10 minutes
Cooking time: 15 minutes
Servings: 5

Ingredients:
2 pounds wings
Juice from 1 lime
1 handful cilantro, chopped
2 garlic cloves, minced
1 jalapeno pepper, chopped
3 tablespoons coconut oil
Salt and black pepper to the taste
Lime wedges for serving
Ranch dip for serving

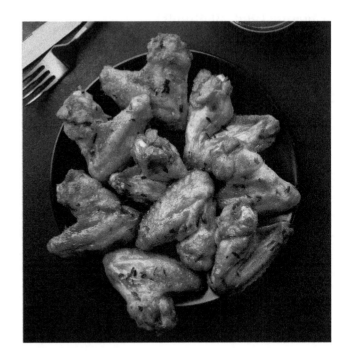

Directions:
1. In a bowl, mix lime juice with cilantro, garlic, jalapeno, coconut oil, salt and pepper and whisk well.
2. Add chicken wings, toss to coat and keep in the fridge for 2 hours.
3. Place chicken wings on your preheated grill over medium high heat and cook for 7 minutes on each side.
4. Serve these amazing chicken wings with ranch did and lime wedges on the side.
Enjoy!

Nutrition: calories 132, fat 5, fiber 1, carbs 4, protein 12

Easy Baked Chicken

Preparation time: 10 minutes
Cooking time: 20 minutes
Servings: 4

Ingredients:
4 bacon strips
4 chicken breasts
3 green onions, chopped
4 ounces ranch dressing
1 ounce coconut aminos
2 tablespoons coconut oil
4 ounces cheddar cheese, grated

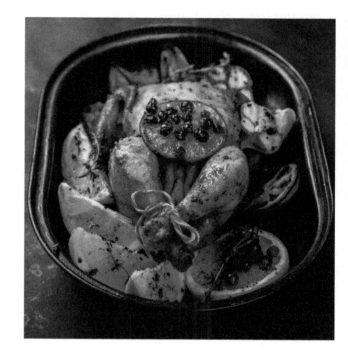

Directions:
1. Heat up a pan with the oil over high heat, add chicken breasts, cook for 7 minutes, flip and cook for 7 more minutes.
2. Meanwhile, heat up another pan over medium high heat, add bacon, cook until it's crispy, transfer to paper towels, drain grease and crumble.
3. Transfer chicken breast to a baking dish, add coconut aminos, crumbled bacon, cheese and green onions on top, introduce in your oven, set on broiler and cook at a high temperature for 5 minutes more.
4. Divide between plates and serve hot.
Enjoy!

Nutrition: calories 450, fat 24, fiber 0, carbs 3, protein 60

Special Italian Chicken

Preparation time: 10 minutes
Cooking time: 20 minutes
Servings: 4

Ingredients:
¼ cup olive oil
1 red onion, chopped
4 chicken breasts, skinless and boneless
4 garlic cloves, minced
Salt and black pepper to the taste
½ cup Italian olives, pitted and chopped
4 anchovy fillets, chopped
1 tablespoon capers, chopped
1 pound tomatoes, chopped
½ teaspoon red chili flakes

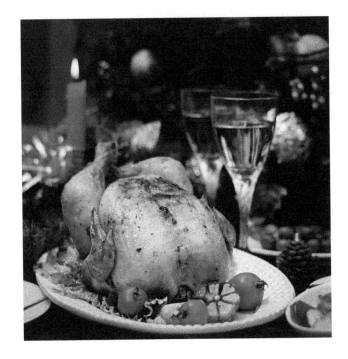

Directions:
1. Season chicken with salt and pepper and rub with half of the oil.
2. Place into a pan which you've heated over high temperature, cook for 2 minutes, flip and cook for 2 minutes more.
3. Introduce chicken breasts in the oven at 450 degrees F and bake for 8 minutes.
4. Take chicken out of the oven and divide between plates.
5. Heat up the same pan with the rest of the oil over medium heat, add capers, onion, garlic, olives, anchovies, chili flakes and
capers, stir and cook for 1 minute.
6. Add salt, pepper and tomatoes, stir and cook for 2 minutes more.
7. Drizzle this over chicken breasts and serve.
Enjoy!

Nutrition: calories 400, fat 20, fiber 1, carbs 2, protein 7

Simple Lemon Chicken

Preparation time: 10 minutes
Cooking time: 45 minutes
Servings: 6

Ingredients:
1 whole chicken, cut into medium pieces
Salt and black pepper to the taste
Juice from 2 lemons
Zest from 2 lemons
Lemon rinds from 2 lemons

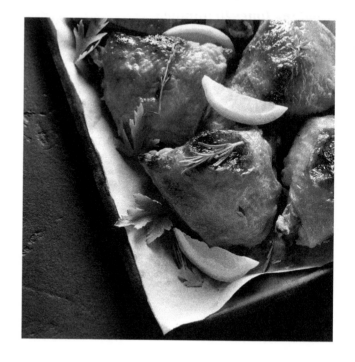

Directions:
1. Put chicken pieces in a baking dish, season with salt and pepper to the taste and drizzle lemon juice.
2. Toss to coat well, add lemon zest and lemon rinds, introduce in the oven at 375 degrees F and bake for 45 minutes.
3. Discard lemon rinds, divide chicken between plates, drizzle sauce from the baking dish over it and serve.
Enjoy!

Nutrition: calories 334, fat 24, fiber 2, carbs 4.5, protein 27

Fried Chicken And Paprika Sauce

Preparation time: 10 minutes
Cooking time: 20 minutes
Servings: 5

Ingredients:
1 tablespoon coconut oil
3 and ½ pounds chicken breasts
1 cup chicken stock
1 and ¼ cups yellow onion, chopped
1 tablespoon lime juice
¼ cup coconut milk
2 teaspoons paprika
1 teaspoon red pepper flakes
2 tablespoons green onions, chopped
Salt and black pepper to the taste

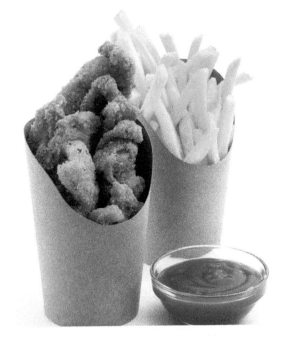

Directions:
1. Heat up a pan with the oil over medium high heat, add chicken, cook for 2 minutes on each side, transfer to a plate and leave aside.
2. Reduce heat to medium, add onions to the pan and cook for 4 minutes.
3. Add stock, coconut milk, pepper flakes, paprika, lime juice, salt and pepper and stir well.
4. Return chicken to the pan, add more salt and pepper, cover pan and cook for 15 minutes.
5. Divide between plates and serve.
Enjoy!

Nutrition: calories 140, fat 4, fiber 3, carbs 3, protein 6

Amazing Chicken Fajitas

Preparation time: 10 minutes
Cooking time: 15 minutes
Servings: 4

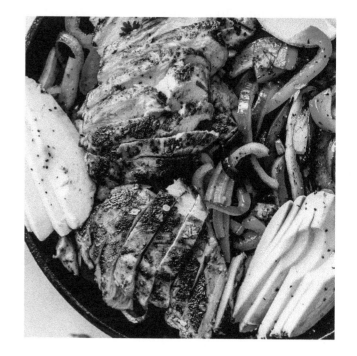

Ingredients:
2 pounds chicken breasts, skinless, boneless and cut into strips
1 teaspoon garlic powder
1 teaspoon chili powder
2 teaspoons cumin
2 tablespoons lime juice
Salt and black pepper to the taste
1 teaspoon sweet paprika
2 tablespoons coconut oil
1 teaspoon coriander, ground
1 green bell pepper, sliced
1 red bell pepper, sliced
1 yellow onion, sliced
1 tablespoon cilantro, chopped
1 avocado, pitted, peeled and sliced
2 limes, cut into wedges

Directions:
1. In a bowl, mix lime juice with chili powder, cumin, salt, pepper, garlic powder, paprika and coriander and stir.
2. Add chicken pieces and toss to coat well.
3. Heat up a pan with half of the oil over medium high heat, add chicken, cook for 3 minutes on each side and transfer to a bowl.
4. Heat up the pan with the rest of the oil over medium heat, add onion and all bell peppers, stir and cook for 6 minutes.
5. Return chicken to pan, add more salt and pepper, stir and divide between plates.
6. Top with avocado, lime wedges and cilantro and serve.
Enjoy!

Nutrition: calories 240, fat 10, fiber 2, carbs 5, protein 20

Skillet Chicken And Mushrooms

Preparation time: 10 minutes
Cooking time: 30 minutes
Servings: 4

Ingredients:
4 chicken thighs
2 cups mushrooms, sliced
¼ cup ghee
Salt and black pepper to the taste
½ teaspoon onion powder
½ teaspoon garlic powder
½ cup water
1 teaspoon Dijon mustard
1 tablespoon tarragon, chopped

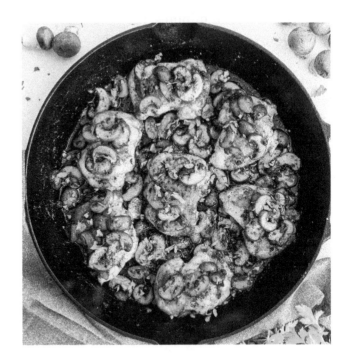

Directions:
1. Heat up a pan with half of the ghee over medium high heat, add chicken thighs, season them with salt, pepper, garlic powder and onion powder, cook the for 3 minutes on each side and transfer to a bowl.
2. Heat up the same pan with the rest of the ghee over medium high heat, add mushrooms, stir and cook for 5 minutes.
3. Add mustard and water and stir well.
4. Return chicken pieces to the pan, stir, cover and cook for 15 minutes.
5. Add tarragon, stir, cook for 5 minutes, divide between plates and serve.
Enjoy!

Nutrition: calories 453, fat 32, fiber 6, carbs 1, protein 36

Chicken And Olives Tapenade

Preparation time: 10 minutes
Cooking time: 10 minutes
Servings: 2

Ingredients:
1 chicken breast cut into 4 pieces
2 tablespoons coconut oil
3 garlic cloves, crushed
½ cup olives tapenade
For the tapenade:
1 cup black olives, pitted
Salt and black pepper to the taste
2 tablespoons olive oil
¼ cup parsley, chopped
1 tablespoons lemon juice

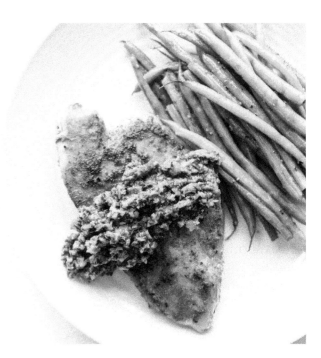

Directions:
1. In your food processor, mix olives with salt, pepper, 2 tablespoons olive oil, lemon juice and parsley, blend very well and transfer to a bowl.
2. Heat up a pan with the coconut oil over medium heat, add garlic, stir and cook for 2 minutes.
3. Add chicken pieces and cook for 4 minutes on each side.
4. Divide chicken on plates and top with the olives tapenade.
Enjoy!

Nutrition: calories 130, fat 12, fiber 0, carbs 3, protein 20

Delicious Duck Breast

Preparation time: 10 minutes
Cooking time: 20 minutes
Servings: 1

Ingredients:
1 medium duck breast, skin scored
1 tablespoon swerve
1 tablespoon heavy cream
2 tablespoons ghee
½ teaspoon orange extract
Salt and black pepper to the taste
1 cup baby spinach
¼ teaspoon sage

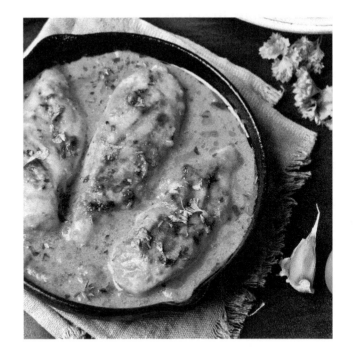

Directions:
1. Heat up a pan with the ghee over medium heat.
2. Once it melts, add swerve and stir until ghee browns.
3. Add orange extract and sage, stir and cook for 2 minutes more.
4. Add heavy cream and stir again.
5. Meanwhile, heat up another pan over medium high heat, add duck breast, skin side down, cook for 4 minutes, flip and cook for another 3 minutes.
6. Pour orange sauce over duck breast, stir and cook for a few minutes more.
7. Add spinach to the pan where you've made the sauce, stir and cook for 1 minute.
8. Take duck off heat, slice duck breast and arrange on a plate.
9. Drizzle the orange sauce on top and serve with the spinach on the side.
Enjoy!

Nutrition: calories 567, fat 56, fiber 0, carbs 0, protein 35

Duck Breast With Tasty Veggies

Preparation time: 10 minutes
Cooking time: 10 minutes
Servings: 2

Ingredients:
2 duck breasts, skin on and thinly sliced
2 zucchinis, sliced
1 tablespoon coconut oil
1 spring onion stack, chopped
1 daikon, chopped
2 green bell peppers, chopped
Salt and black pepper to the taste

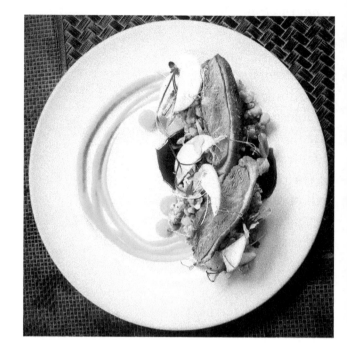

Directions:
1. Heat up a pan with the oil over medium high heat, add spring onions, stir and cook for 2 minutes.
2. Add zucchinis, daikon, bell peppers, salt and pepper, stir and cook for 10 minutes more.
3. Heat up another pan over medium high heat, add duck slices, cook for 3 minutes on each side and transfer to the pan with the veggies.
4. Cook everything for 3 minutes more, divide between plates and serve.
Enjoy!

Nutrition: calories 450, fat 23, fiber 3, carbs 8, protein 50

Duck Breast Salad

Preparation time: 10 minutes
Cooking time: 15 minutes
Servings: 4

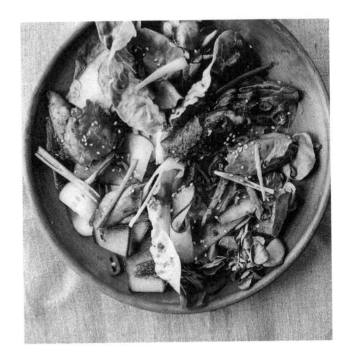

Ingredients:
1 tablespoon swerve
1 shallot, chopped
¼ cup red vinegar
¼ cup olive oil
¼ cup water
¾ cup raspberries
1 tablespoon Dijon mustard
Salt and black pepper to the taste
For the salad:
10 ounces baby spinach
2 medium duck breasts, boneless
4 ounces goat cheese, crumbled
Salt and black pepper to the taste
½ pint raspberries
½ cup pecans halves

Directions:
1. In your blender, mix swerve with shallot, vinegar, water, oil, ¾ cup raspberries, mustard, salt and pepper and blend very well.
2. Strain this, put into a bowl and leave aside.
3. Score duck breast, season with salt and pepper and place skin side down into a pan heated up over medium high heat.
4. Cook for 8 minutes, flip and cook for 5 minutes more.
5. Divide spinach on plates, sprinkle goat cheese, pecan halves and ½ pint raspberries.
6. Slice duck breasts and add on top of raspberries.
7. Drizzle the raspberries vinaigrette on top and serve.
Enjoy!

Nutrition: calories 455, fat 40, fiber 4, carbs 6, protein 18

Turkey Pie

Preparation time: 10 minutes
Cooking time: 40 minutes
Servings: 6

Ingredients:
2 cups turkey stock
1 cup turkey meat, cooked and shredded
Salt and black pepper to the taste
1 teaspoon thyme, chopped
½ cup kale, chopped
½ cup butternut squash, peeled and chopped
½ cup cheddar cheese, shredded
¼ teaspoon paprika
¼ teaspoon garlic powder
¼ teaspoon xanthan gum
Cooking spray
For the crust:, ¼ cup ghee
¼ teaspoon xanthan gum, 2 cups almond flour
A pinch of salt, 1 egg, ¼ cup cheddar cheese

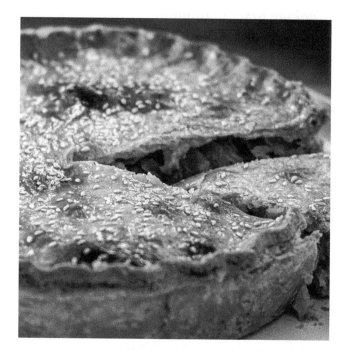

Directions:
1. Heat up a pot with the stock over medium heat.
2. Add squash and turkey meat, stir and cook for 10 minutes.
3. Add garlic powder, kale, thyme, paprika, salt, pepper and ½ cup cheddar cheese and stir well.
4. In a bowl, mix ¼ teaspoon xanthan gum with ½ cup stock from the pot, stir well and add everything to the pot.
5. Take off heat and leave aside for now.
6. In a bowl, mix flour with ¼ teaspoon xanthan gum and a pinch of salt and stir.
7. Add ghee, egg and ¼ cup cheddar cheese and stir everything until you obtain your pie crust dough.
8. Shape a ball and keep in the fridge for now.
9. Spray a baking dish with cooking spray and spread pie filling on the bottom.
10. Transfer dough to a working surface, roll into a circle and top filling with this.
11. Press well and seal edges, introduce in the oven at 350 degrees F and bake for 35 minutes.
12. Leave the pie to cool down a bit and serve
Enjoy!

Nutrition: calories 320, fat 23, fiber 8, carbs 6, protein 16.

Turkey Soup

Preparation time: 10 minutes
Cooking time: 30 minutes
Servings: 4

Ingredients:
3 celery stalks, chopped
1 yellow onion, chopped
1 tablespoon ghee
6 cups turkey stock
Salt and black pepper to the taste
¼ cup parsley, chopped
3 cups baked spaghetti squash, chopped
3 cups turkey, cooked and shredded

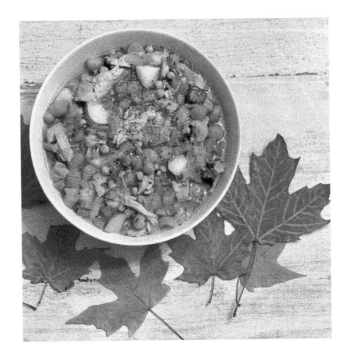

Directions:
1. Heat up a pot with the ghee over medium high heat, add celery and onion, stir and cook for 5 minutes.
2. Add parsley, stock, turkey meat, salt and pepper, stir and cook for 20 minutes.
3. Add spaghetti squash, stir and cook turkey soup for 10 minutes more.
4. Divide into bowls and serve.
Enjoy!

Nutrition: calories 150, fat 4, fiber 1, carbs 3, protein 10

Baked Turkey Delight

Preparation time: 10 minutes
Cooking time: 45 minutes
Servings: 8

Ingredients:
4 cups zucchinis, cut with a spiralizer
1 egg, whisked
3 cups cabbage, shredded
3 cups turkey meat, cooked and shredded
½ cup turkey stock
½ cup cream cheese
1 teaspoon poultry seasoning
2 cup cheddar cheese, grated
½ cup parmesan cheese, grated
Salt and black pepper to the taste
¼ teaspoon garlic powder

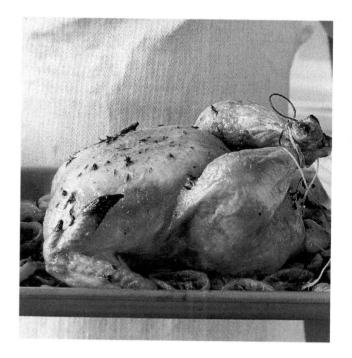

Directions:
1. Heat up a pan with the stock over medium-low heat.
2. Add egg, cream, parmesan, cheddar cheese, salt, pepper, poultry seasoning and garlic powder, stir and bring to a gentle simmer.
3. Add turkey meat and cabbage, stir and take off heat.
4. Place zucchini noodles in a baking dish, add some salt and pepper, pour turkey mix and spread.
5. Cover with tin foil, introduce in the oven at 400 degrees F and bake for 35 minutes.
6. Leave aside to cool down a bit before serving.
Enjoy!

Nutrition: calories 240, fat 15, fiber 1, carbs 3, protein 25

Delicious Turkey Chili

Preparation time: 10 minutes
Cooking time: 20 minutes
Servings: 8

Ingredients:
4 cups turkey meat, cooked and shredded
2 cups squash, chopped
6 cups chicken stock
Salt and black pepper to the taste
1 tablespoon canned chipotle peppers, chopped
½ teaspoon garlic powder
½ cup salsa verde
1 teaspoon coriander, ground
2 teaspoons cumin, ground
¼ cup sour cream
1 tablespoon cilantro, chopped

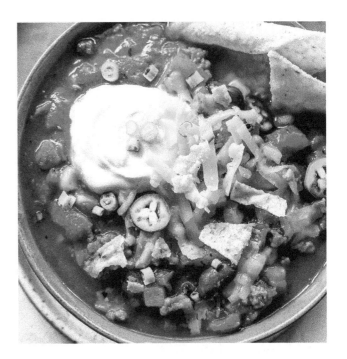

Directions:
1. Heat up a pan with the stock over medium heat.
2. Add squash, stir and cook for 10 minutes.
3. Add turkey, chipotles, garlic powder, salsa verde, cumin, coriander, salt and pepper, stir and cook for 10 minutes.
4. Add sour cream, stir, take off heat and divide into bowls.
5. Top with some chopped cilantro and serve.
Enjoy!

Nutrition: calories 154, fat 5, fiber 3, carbs 2, protein 27

Turkey And Tomato Curry

Preparation time: 10 minutes
Cooking time: 20 minutes
Servings: 4

Ingredients:
18 ounces turkey meat, minced
3 ounces spinach
20 ounces canned tomatoes, chopped
2 tablespoons coconut oil
2 tablespoons coconut cream
2 garlic cloves, minced
2 yellow onions, sliced
1 tablespoon coriander, ground
2 tablespoons ginger, grated
1 tablespoons turmeric
1 tablespoon cumin, ground
Salt and black pepper to the taste
2 tablespoons chili powder

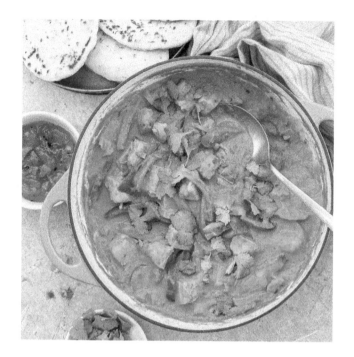

Directions:
1. Heat up a pan with the coconut oil over medium heat, add onion, stir and cook for 5 minutes.
2. Add ginger and garlic, stir and cook for 1 minute.
3. Add tomatoes, salt, pepper, coriander, cumin, turmeric and chili powder and stir.
4. Add coconut cream, stir and cook for 10 minutes.
5. Blend using an immersion blender and mix with spinach and turkey meat.
6. Bring to a simmer, cook for 15 minutes more and serve.
Enjoy!

Nutrition: calories 240, fat 4, fiber 3, carbs 2, protein 12

Turkey And Cranberry Salad

Preparation time: 10 minutes
Cooking time: 0 minutes
Servings: 4

Ingredients:
4 cups romaine lettuce leaves, torn
2 cups turkey breast, cooked and cubed
1 orange, peeled and cut into small segments
1 red apple, cored and chopped
3 tablespoons walnuts, chopped
3 kiwis, peeled and sliced
¼ cup cranberries
1 cup cranberry sauce
1 cup orange juice

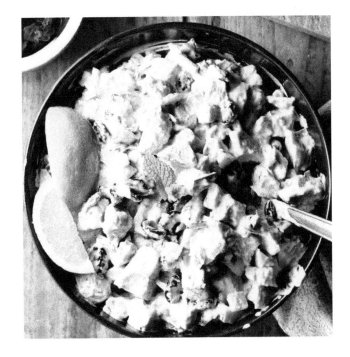

Directions:
1. In a salad bowl, mix lettuce with turkey, orange segments, apple pieces, cranberries and walnut and toss to coat.
2. In another bowl, mix cranberry sauce and orange juice and stir.
3. Drizzle this over turkey salad, toss to coat and serve with kiwis on top.
Enjoy!

Nutrition: calories 120, fat 2, fiber 1, carbs 3, protein 7

Stuffed Chicken Breast

Preparation time: 10 minutes
Cooking time: 15 minutes
Servings: 3

Ingredients:
8 ounces spinach, cooked and chopped
3 chicken breasts
Salt and black pepper to the taste
4 ounces cream cheese, soft
3 ounces feta cheese, crumbled
1 garlic clove, minced
1 tablespoon coconut oil

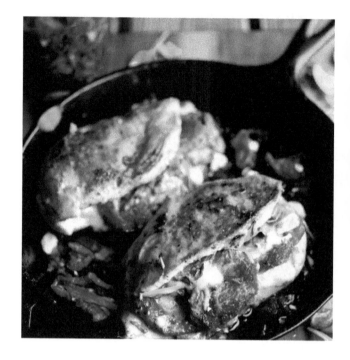

Directions:
1. In a bowl, mix feta cheese with cream cheese, spinach, salt, pepper and the garlic and stir well.
2. Place chicken breasts on a working surface, cut a pocket in each, stuff them with the spinach mix and season them with
salt and pepper to the taste.
3. Heat up a pan with the oil over medium high heat, add stuffed chicken, cook for 5 minutes on each side and then introduce everything in the oven at 450 degrees F.
4. Bake for 10 minutes, divide between plates and serve.
Enjoy!

Nutrition: calories 290, fat 12, fiber 2, carbs 4, protein 24

Chicken And Mustard Sauce

Preparation time: 10 minutes
Cooking time: 30 minutes
Servings: 3

Ingredients:
8 bacon strips, chopped
1/3 cup Dijon mustard
Salt and black pepper to the taste
1 cup yellow onion, chopped
1 tablespoon olive oil
1 and ½ cups chicken stock
3 chicken breasts, skinless and boneless
¼ teaspoon sweet paprika

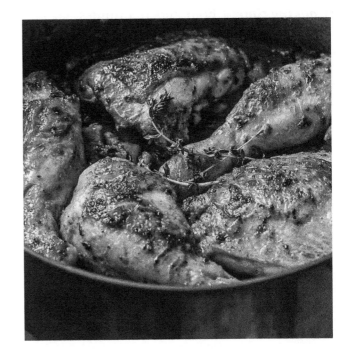

Directions:
1. In a bowl, mix paprika with mustard, salt and pepper and stir well.
2. Spread this on chicken breasts and massage.
3. Heat up a pan over medium high heat, add bacon, stir, cook until it browns and transfer to a plate.
4. Heat up the same pan with the oil over medium high heat, add chicken breasts, cook for 2 minutes on each side and also
transfer to a plate.
5. Heat up the pan once again over medium high heat, add stock, stir and bring to a simmer.
6. Add bacon and onions, salt and pepper and stir.
7. Return chicken to pan as well, stir gently and simmer over medium heat for 20 minutes, turning meat halfway.
8. Divide chicken on plates, drizzle the sauce over it and serve.
Enjoy!

Nutrition: calories 223, fat 8, fiber 1, carbs 3, protein 26

Delicious Salsa Chicken

Preparation time: 10 minutes
Cooking time: 1 hour and 15 minutes
Servings: 6

Ingredients:
6 chicken breasts, skinless and boneless
2 cups jarred salsa
Salt and black pepper to the taste
1 cup cheddar cheese, shredded
Vegetable cooking spray

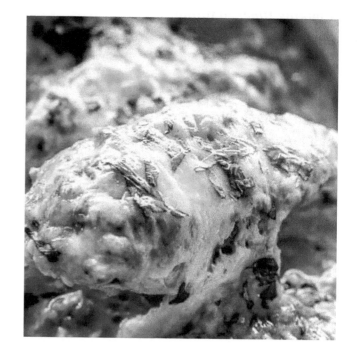

Directions:
1. Spray a baking dish with cooking oil, place chicken breasts on it, season with salt and pepper and pour salsa all over.
2. Introduce in the oven at 425 degrees F and bake for 1 hour.
3. Spread cheese and bake for 15 minutes more.
4. Divide between plates and serve.
Enjoy!

Nutrition: calories 120, fat 2, fiber 2, carbs 6, protein 10

Delicious Italian Chicken

Preparation time: 10 minutes
Cooking time: 1 hour
Servings: 6

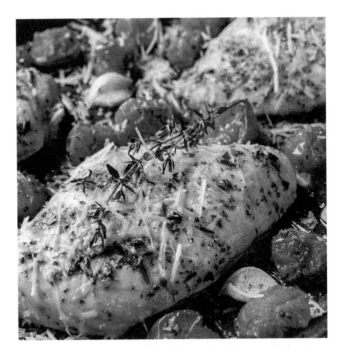

Ingredients:
8 ounces mushrooms, chopped
1 pound Italian sausage, chopped
2 tablespoons avocado oil
6 cherry peppers, chopped
1 red bell pepper, chopped
1 red onion, sliced
2 tablespoons garlic, minced
2 cups cherry tomatoes, halved
4 chicken thighs
Salt and black pepper to the taste
½ cup chicken stock
1 tablespoon balsamic vinegar
2 teaspoons oregano, dried
Some chopped parsley for serving

Directions:
1. Heat up a pan with half of the oil over medium heat, add sausages, stir, brown for a few minutes and transfer to a plate.
2. Heat up the pan again with the rest of the oil over medium heat, add chicken thighs, season with salt and pepper, cook for 3 minutes on each side and transfer to a plate.
3. Heat up the pan again over medium heat, add cherry peppers, mushrooms, onion and bell pepper, stir and cook for 4 minutes.
4. Add garlic, stir and cook for 2 minutes.
5. Add stock, vinegar, salt, pepper, oregano and cherry tomatoes and stir.
6. Add chicken pieces and sausages ones, stir gently, transfer everything to the oven at 400 degrees and bake for 30 minutes.
7. Sprinkle parsley, divide between plates and serve.
Enjoy!

Nutrition: calories 340, fat 33, fiber 3, carbs 4, protein 20

Chicken Casserole

Preparation time: 10 minutes
Cooking time: 40 minutes
Servings: 8

Ingredients:
1 and ½ pounds chicken breast, skinless and boneless and cubed
Salt and black pepper to the taste
1 egg
1 cup almond flour
¼ cup parmesan, grated
½ teaspoon garlic powder
1 and ½ teaspoons parsley, dried
½ teaspoon basil, dried
4 tablespoons avocado oil
4 cups spaghetti squash, already cooked
6 ounces mozzarella, shredded
1 and ½ cups keto marinara sauce
Fresh basil, chopped for serving

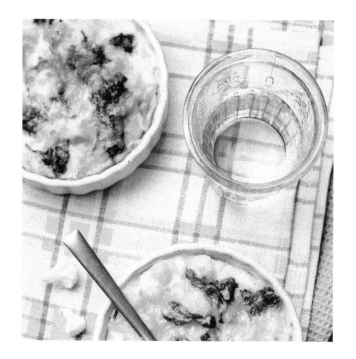

Directions:
1. In a bowl, mix almond flour with parm, salt, pepper, garlic powder and 1 teaspoon parsley and stir.
2. In another bowl, whisk the egg with a pinch of salt and pepper.
3. Dip chicken in egg and then in almond flour mix.
4. Heat up a pan with 3 tablespoons oil over medium high heat, add chicken, cook until they are golden on both sides and transfer to paper towels.
5. In a bowl, mix spaghetti squash with salt, pepper, dried basil, 1 tablespoon oil and the rest of the parsley and stir.
6. Spread this into a heatproof dish, add chicken pieces and then the marinara sauce.
7. Top with shredded mozzarella, introduce in the oven at 375 degrees F and bake for 30 minutes.
8. Sprinkle fresh basil at the end, leave casserole aside to cool
down a bit, divide between plates and serve.
Enjoy!

Nutrition: calories 300, fat 6, fiber 3, carbs 5, protein 28

Chicken Stuffed Peppers

Preparation time: 10 minutes
Cooking time: 40 minutes
Servings: 3

Ingredients:
2 cups cauliflower florets
Salt and black pepper to the taste
1 small yellow onion, chopped
2 chicken breasts, skinless, boneless, cooked
and shredded
2 tablespoons fajita seasoning
1 tablespoon ghee
6 bell peppers, tops cut off and seeds removed
2/3 cup water

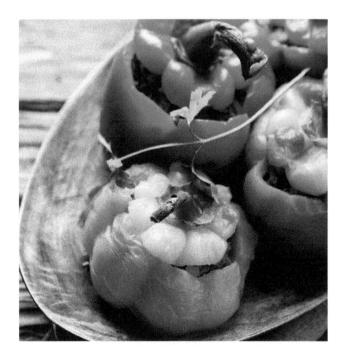

Directions:
1. Put cauliflower florets in your food processor, add a pinch of salt and pepper, pulse well and transfer to a bowl.
2. Heat up a pan with the ghee over medium heat, add onions, stir and cook for 2 minutes.
3. Add cauliflower, stir and cook for 3 minutes more.
4. Add seasoning, salt, pepper, water and chicken, stir and cook for 2 minutes.
5. Place bell peppers on a lined baking sheet, stuff each with chicken mix, introduce in the oven at 350 degrees F and bake
for 30 minutes.
6. Divide them between plates and serve.
Enjoy!

Nutrition: calories 200, fat 6, fiber 3, carbs 6, protein 14

Creamy Chicken

Preparation time: 10 minutes
Cooking time: 1 hour
Servings: 4

Ingredients:
4 chicken breasts, skinless and boneless
½ cup mayo
½ cup sour cream
Salt and black pepper to the taste
¾ cup parmesan, grated
Cooking spray
8 mozzarella slices
1 teaspoon garlic powder

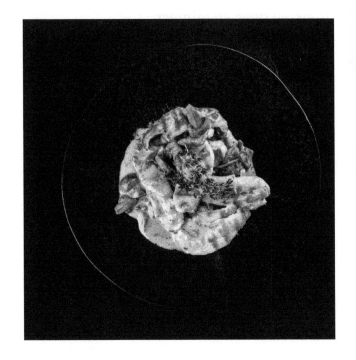

Directions:
1. Spray a baking dish, place chicken breasts in it and top each piece with 2 mozzarella slices.
2. In a bowl, mix parm with salt, pepper, mayo, garlic powder and sour cream and stir well.
3. Spread this over chicken, introduce dish in the oven at 375 degrees F and bake for 1 hour.
4. Divide between plates and serve.
Enjoy!

Nutrition: calories 240, fat 4, fiber 3, carbs 6, protein 20

Different Chicken Casserole

Preparation time: 10 minutes
Cooking time: 45 minutes
Servings: 4

Ingredients:
3 cups cheddar cheese, grated
10 ounces broccoli florets
3 chicken breasts, skinless, boneless, cooked and cubed
1 cup mayo
1 tablespoon coconut oil, melted
1/3 cup chicken stock
Salt and black pepper to the taste
Juice of 1 lemon

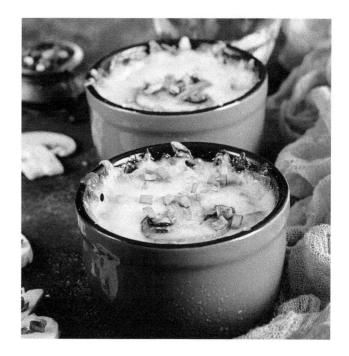

Directions:
1. Grease a baking dish with oil and arrange chicken pieces on the bottom.
2. Spread broccoli florets and then half of the cheese.
3. In a bowl, mix mayo with stock, salt, pepper and lemon juice.
4. Pour this over chicken, sprinkle the rest of the cheese, cover dish with tin foil and bake in the oven at 350 degrees F for 30 minutes
5. Remove foil and bake for 20 minutes more.
6. Serve hot.
Enjoy!

Nutrition: calories 250, fat 5, fiber 4, carbs 6, protein 25

Creamy Chicken Soup

Preparation time: 10 minutes
Cooking time: 20 minutes
Servings: 4

Ingredients:
3 tablespoons ghee
4 ounces cream cheese
2 cups chicken meat, cooked and shredded
1/3 cup red sauce
4 cups chicken stock
Salt and black pepper to the taste
½ cup sour cream
¼ cup celery, chopped

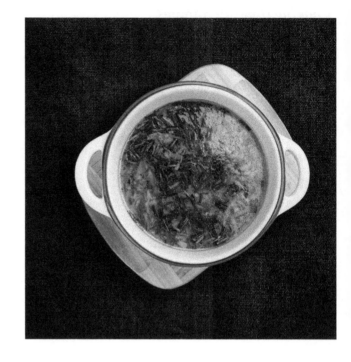

Directions:
1. In your blender, mix stock with red sauce, cream cheese, ghee, salt, pepper and sour cream and pulse well.
2. Transfer this to a pot, heat up over medium heat and add celery and chicken.
3. Stir, simmer for a few minutes, divide into bowls and serve.
Enjoy!

Nutrition: calories 400, fat 23, fiber 5, carbs 5, protein 30

Amazing Chicken Crepes

Preparation time: 10 minutes
Cooking time: 30 minutes
Servings: 8

Ingredients:
6 eggs
6 ounces cream cheese, 1 teaspoon erythritol
1 and ½ tablespoons coconut flour
1/3 cup parmesan, grated
A pinch of xanthan gum
Cooking spray
For the filling:
8 ounces spinach, 8 ounces mushrooms, sliced
8 ounces rotisserie chicken, shredded
8 ounces cheese blend, 2 ounces cream cheese
1 garlic clove, minced
1 small yellow onion, chopped
Liquids:
2 tablespoons red wine vinegar, 2 tablespoons ghee, ½ cup heavy cream, 1 teaspoon Worcestershire sauce, ¼ cup chicken stock, A pinch of nutmeg, Chopped parsley, Salt and black pepper to the taste

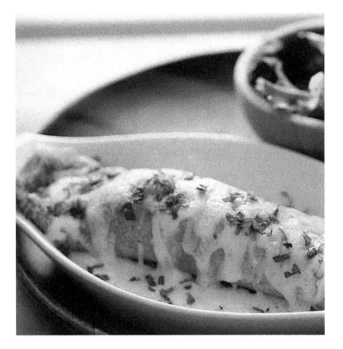

Directions:
1. In a bowl, mix 6 ounces cream cheese with eggs, parm, erythritol, xanthan and coconut flour and stir very well until you obtain a crepes batter.
2. Heat up a pan over medium heat, spray some cooking oil, pour some of the batters, spread well into the pan, cook for 2 minutes, flip and cook for 30 seconds more.
3. Repeat with the rest of the batter and place all crepes on a plate.
4. Heat up a pan with 2 tablespoon ghee over medium high heat, add onion, stir and cook for 2 minutes. Add garlic, stir and cook for 1 minute more. Add mushrooms, stir and cook for 2 minutes.. Add chicken, spinach, salt, pepper, stock, vinegar, nutmeg, Worcestershire sauce, heavy cream, 2 ounces cream cheese and ounce cheese blend, stir everything and cook for 7 minutes more. Fill each crepe with this mix, roll them and arrange them all in a baking dish.
5. Top with 2 ounces cheese blend, introduce in preheated broiler for a couple of minutes.
6. Divide crepes on plates, top with chopped parsley and serve.
Enjoy!

Nutrition: calories 360, fat 32, fiber 2, carbs 7, protein 20

Unbelievable Chicken Dish

Preparation time: 10 minutes
Cooking time: 50 minutes
Servings: 4

Ingredients:
3 pounds chicken breasts
2 ounces muenster cheese, cubed
2 ounces cream cheese
4 ounces cheddar cheese, cubed
2 ounces provolone cheese, cubed
1 zucchini, shredded
Salt and black pepper to the taste
1 teaspoon garlic, minced
½ cup bacon, cooked and crumbled

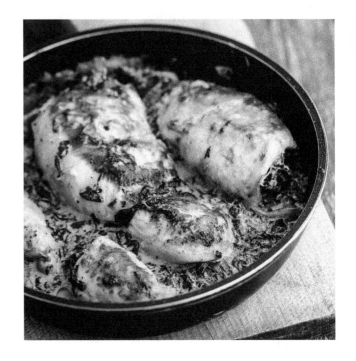

Directions:
1. Season zucchini with salt and pepper, leave aside few minutes, squeeze well and transfer to a bowl.
2. Add bacon, garlic, more salt and pepper, cream cheese, cheddar cheese, muenster cheese and provolone cheese and stir.
3. Cut slits into chicken breasts, season with salt and pepper and stuff with zucchini and cheese mix.
4. Place on a lined baking sheet, introduce in the oven at 400 degrees F and bake for 45 minutes.
5. Divide between plates and serve.
Enjoy!

Nutrition: calories 455, fat 20, fiber 0, carbs 2, protein 57

Delicious Crusted Chicken

Preparation time: 10 minutes
Cooking time: 35 minutes
Servings: 4

Ingredients:
4 bacon slices, cooked and crumbled
4 chicken breasts, skinless and boneless
1 tablespoon water
½ cup avocado oil
1 egg, whisked
Salt and black pepper to the taste
1 cup asiago cheese, shredded
¼ teaspoon garlic powder
1 cup parmesan cheese, grated

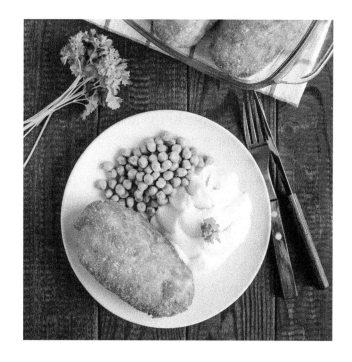

Directions:
1. In a bowl, mix parmesan cheese with garlic, salt and pepper and stir.
2. Put whisked egg in another bowl and mix with the water.
3. Season chicken with salt and pepper and dip each piece into egg and then into cheese mix.
4. Heat up a pan with the oil over medium high heat, add chicken breasts, cook until they are golden on both sides and transfer to a baking pan.
5. Introduce in the oven at 350 degrees F and bake for 20 minutes.
6. Top chicken with bacon and asiago cheese, introduce in the oven, turn on broiler and broil for a couple of minutes.
7. Serve hot.
Enjoy!

Nutrition: calories 400, fat 22, fiber 1, carbs 1, protein 47

Cheesy Chicken

Preparation time: 10 minutes
Cooking time: 30 minutes
Servings: 4

Ingredients:
1 zucchini, chopped
Salt and black pepper to the taste
1 teaspoon garlic powder
1 tablespoon avocado oil
2 chicken breasts, skinless and boneless
and sliced
1 tomato, chopped
½ teaspoon oregano, dried
½ teaspoon basil, dried
½ cup mozzarella cheese, shredded

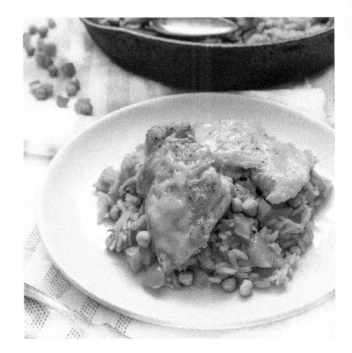

Directions:
1. Season chicken with salt, pepper and garlic powder.
2. Heat up a pan with the oil over medium heat, add chicken slices, brown on all sides and transfer them to a baking dish.
3. Heat up the pan again over medium heat, add zucchini, oregano, tomato, basil, salt and pepper, stir, cook for 2 minutes and pour over chicken.
4. Introduce in the oven at 325 degrees F and bake for 20 minutes.
5. Spread mozzarella over chicken, introduce in the oven again and bake for 5 minutes more.
6. Divide between plates and serve.
Enjoy!

Nutrition: calories 235, fat 4, fiber 1, carbs 2, protein 35

Orange Chicken

Preparation time: 10 minutes
Cooking time: 15 minutes
Servings: 4

Ingredients:
2 pounds chicken thighs, skinless, boneless and cut into pieces
Salt and black pepper to the taste
3 tablespoons coconut oil
¼ cup coconut flour
For the sauce:
2 tablespoons fish sauce
1 and ½ teaspoons orange extract
1 tablespoon ginger, grated
¼ cup orange juice
2 teaspoons stevia, 1 tablespoon orange zest
¼ teaspoon sesame seeds
2 tablespoons scallions, chopped
½ teaspoon coriander, ground
1 cup water, ¼ teaspoon red pepper flakes
2 tablespoons gluten free soy sauce

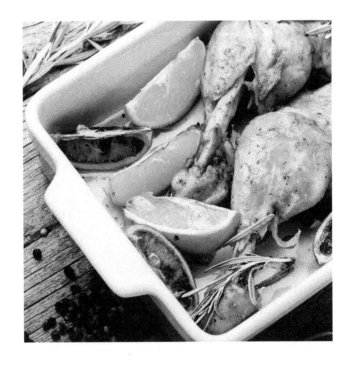

Directions:
1. In a bowl, mix coconut flour and salt and pepper and stir.
2. Add chicken pieces and toss to coat well.
3. Heat up a pan with the oil over medium heat, add chicken, cook until they are golden on both sides and transfer to a bowl.
4. In your blender, mix orange juice with ginger, fish sauce, soy sauce, stevia, orange extract, water and coriander and blend
well.
5. Pour this into a pan and heat up over medium heat.
6. Add chicken, stir and cook for 2 minutes.
7. Add sesame seeds, orange zest, scallions and pepper flakes, stir cook for 2 minutes and take off heat.
8. Divide between plates and serve.
Enjoy!

Nutrition: calories 423, fat 20, fiber 5, carbs 6, protein 45

Chicken Pie

Preparation time: 10 minutes
Cooking time: 45 minutes
Servings: 4

Ingredients:
½ cup yellow onion, chopped
3 tablespoons ghee
½ cup carrots, chopped, 3 garlic cloves, minced
Salt and black pepper to the taste
¾ cup heavy cream
½ cup chicken stock
12 ounces chicken, cubed
2 tablespoons Dijon mustard
¾ cup cheddar cheese, shredded
For the dough:
¾ cup almond flour
3 tablespoons cream cheese
1 and ½ cup mozzarella cheese, shredded
1 egg, 1 teaspoon onion powder
1 teaspoon garlic powder
1 teaspoon Italian seasoning
Salt and black pepper to the taste

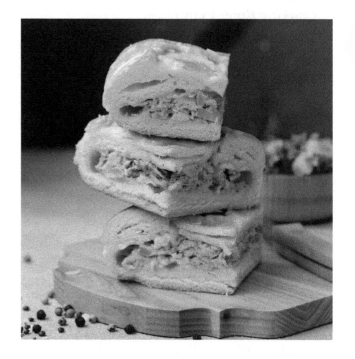

Directions:
1. Heat up a pan with the ghee over medium heat, add onion, carrots, garlic, salt and pepper, stir and cook for 5 minutes. Add chicken, stir and cook for 3 minutes more.
2. Add heavy cream, stock, salt, pepper and mustard, stir and cook for 7 minutes more.
3. Add cheddar cheese, stir well, take off heat and keep warm.
4. Meanwhile, in a bowl, mix mozzarella with cream cheese, stir and heat up in your microwave for 1 minute. Add garlic powder, Italian seasoning, salt, pepper, onion powder, flour and egg and stir well. Knead your dough very well, divide into 4 pieces and flatten each into a circle.
5. Divide chicken mix into 4 ramekins, top each with a dough circle, introduce in the oven at 375 degrees F for 25 minutes.
6. Serve your chicken pies warm.
Enjoy!

Nutrition: calories 600, fat 54, fiber 14, carbs 10, protein 45

Bacon Wrapped Chicken

Preparation time: 10 minutes
Cooking time: 35 minutes
Servings: 4

Ingredients:
1 tablespoon chives, chopped
8 ounces cream cheese
2 pounds chicken breasts,
skinless and boneless
12 bacon slices
Salt and black pepper to the taste

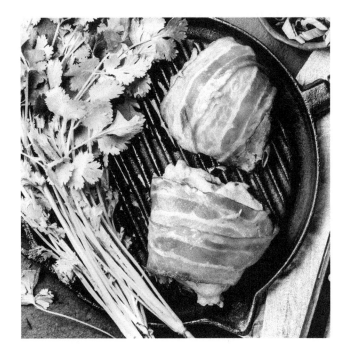

Directions:
1. Heat up a pan over medium heat, add bacon, cook until it's half done, transfer to paper towels and drain grease.
2. In a bowl, mix cream cheese with salt, pepper and chives and stir.
3. Use a meat tenderizer to flatten chicken breasts well, divide cream cheese mix, roll them up and wrap each in a cooked bacon slice.
4. Arrange wrapped chicken breasts into a baking dish, introduce in the oven at 375 degrees F and bake for 30 minutes.
5. Divide between plates and serve.
Enjoy!

Nutrition: calories 700, fat 45, fiber 4, carbs 5, protein 45

So Delicious Chicken Wings

Preparation time: 10 minutes
Cooking time: 55 minutes
Servings: 4

Ingredients:
3 pounds chicken wings
Salt and black pepper to the taste
3 tablespoons coconut aminos
2 teaspoons white vinegar
3 tablespoons rice vinegar
3 tablespoons stevia
¼ cup scallions, chopped
½ teaspoon xanthan gum
5 dried chilies, chopped

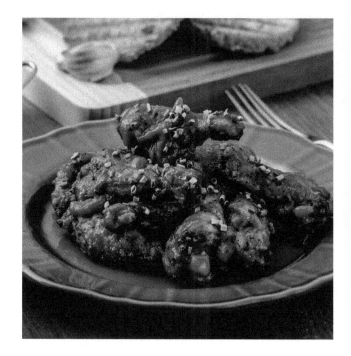

Directions:
1. Spread chicken wings on a lined baking sheet, season with salt and pepper, introduce in the oven at 375 degrees F and bake for
45 minutes.
2. Meanwhile, heat up a small pan over medium heat, add white vinegar, rice vinegar, coconut aminos, stevia, xanthan gum, scallions and chilies, stir well, bring to a boil, cook for 2 minutes and take off heat.
3. Dip chicken wings into this sauce, arrange them all on the baking sheet again and bake for 10 minutes more.
4. Serve them hot.
Enjoy!

Nutrition: calories 415, fat 23, fiber 3, carbs 2, protein 27

Chicken In Creamy Sauce

Preparation time: 10 minutes
Cooking time: 1 hour and 10 minutes
Servings: 4

Ingredients:
8 chicken thighs
Salt and black pepper to the taste
1 yellow onion, chopped
1 tablespoon coconut oil
4 bacon strips, chopped
4 garlic cloves, minced
10 ounces cremini mushrooms, halved
2 cups white chardonnay wine
1 cup whipping cream
A handful parsley, chopped

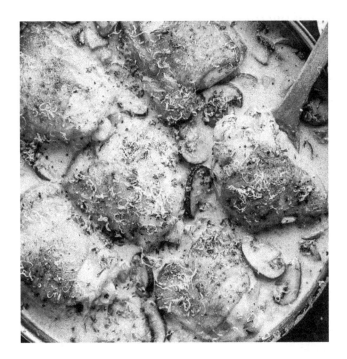

Directions:
1. Heat up a pan with the oil over medium heat, add bacon, stir, cook until it's crispy, take off heat and transfer to paper towels.
2. Heat up the pan with the bacon fat over medium heat, add chicken pieces, season them with salt and pepper, cook until they brown and also transfer to paper towels.
3. Heat up the pan again over medium heat, add onions, stir and cook for 6 minutes.
4. Add garlic, stir, cook for 1 minute and transfer next to bacon pieces.
5. Return pan to stove and heat up again over medium temperature.
6. Add mushrooms stir and cook them for 5 minutes.
7. Return chicken, bacon, garlic and onion to pan.
8. Add wine, stir, bring to a boil, reduce heat and simmer for 40 minutes.
9. Add parsley and cream, stir and cook for 10 minutes more.
10. Divide between plates and serve.
Enjoy!

Nutrition: calories 340, fat 10, fiber 7, carbs 4, protein 24

Delightful Chicken

Preparation time: 10 minutes
Cooking time: 1 hour
Servings: 4

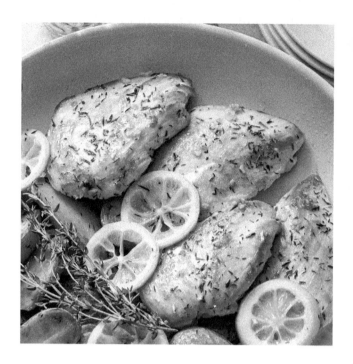

Ingredients:
6 chicken breasts, skinless and boneless
Salt and black pepper to the taste
¼ cup jalapenos, chopped
5 bacon slices, chopped
8 ounces cream cheese
¼ cup yellow onion, chopped
½ cup mayonnaise
½ cup parmesan, grated
1 cup cheddar cheese, grated
For the topping:
2 ounces pork skins, crushed
4 tablespoons melted ghee
½ cup parmesan

Directions:
1. Arrange chicken breasts in a baking dish, season with salt and pepper, introduce in the oven at 425 degrees F and bake for 40 minutes.
2. Meanwhile, heat up a pan over medium heat, add bacon, stir, cook until it's crispy and transfer to a plate.
3. Heat up the pan again over medium heat, add onions, stir and cook for 4 minutes.
4. Take off heat, add bacon, jalapeno, cream cheese, mayo, cheddar cheese and ½ cup parm and stir well..
5. Spread this over chicken.
6. In a bowl, mix pork skin with ghee and ½ cup parm and stir.
7. Spread this over chicken as well, introduce in the oven and bake for 15 minutes more.
8. Serve hot.
Enjoy!

Nutrition: calories 340, fat 12, fiber 2, carbs 5, protein 20

Tasty Chicken And Sour Cream Sauce

Preparation time: 10 minutes
Cooking time: 40 minutes
Servings: 4

Ingredients:
4 chicken thighs
Salt and black pepper to the taste
1 teaspoon onion powder
¼ cup sour cream
2 tablespoons sweet paprika

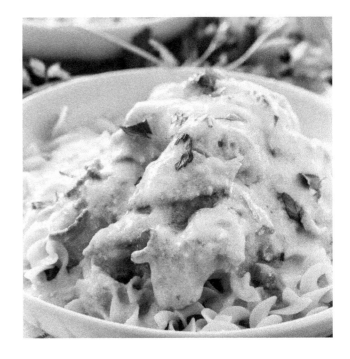

Directions:
1. In a bowl, mix paprika with salt, pepper and onion powder and stir.
2. Season chicken pieces with this paprika mix, arrange them on a lined baking sheet and bake in the oven at 400 degrees F for 40 minutes.
3. Divide chicken on plates and leave aside for now.
4. Pour juices from the pan into a bowl and add sour cream.
5. Stir this sauce very well and drizzle over chicken.
Enjoy!

Nutrition: calories 384, fat 31, fiber 2, carbs 1, protein 33

Tasty Chicken Stroganoff

Preparation time: 10 minutes
Cooking time: 4 hours and 10 minutes
Servings: 4

Ingredients:
2 garlic cloves, minced
8 ounces mushrooms, roughly chopped
¼ teaspoon celery seeds, ground
1 cup chicken stock
1 cup coconut milk
1 yellow onion, chopped
1 pound chicken breasts, cut into medium pieces
1 and ½ teaspoons thyme, dried
2 tablespoons parsley, chopped
Salt and black pepper to the teste
4 zucchinis, cut with a spiralizer

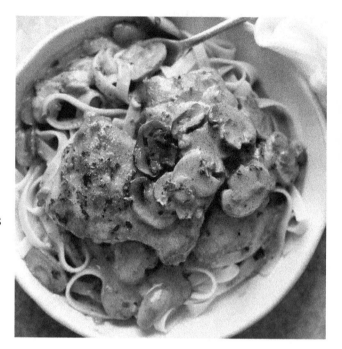

Directions:
1. Put chicken in your slow cooker.
2. Add salt, pepper, onion, garlic, mushrooms, coconut milk, celery seeds, stock, half of the parsley and thyme.
3. Stir, cover and cook on High for 4 hours.
4. Uncover pot, add more salt and pepper if needed and the rest of the parsley and stir.
5. Heat up a pan with water over medium heat, add some salt, bring to a boil, add zucchini pasta, cook for 1 minute and drain.
6. Divide on plates, add chicken mix on top and serve.
Enjoy!

Nutrition: calories 364, fat 22, fiber 2, carbs 4, protein 24

Tasty Chicken Gumbo

Preparation time: 10 minutes
Cooking time: 7 hours
Servings: 5

Ingredients:
2 sausages, sliced
3 chicken breasts, cubed
2 tablespoons oregano, dried
2 bell peppers, chopped
1 small yellow onion, chopped
28 ounces canned tomatoes, chopped
3 tablespoons thyme, dried
2 tablespoons garlic powder
2 tablespoons mustard powder
1 teaspoon cayenne powder
1 tablespoons chili powder
Salt and black pepper to the taste
6 tablespoons Creole seasoning

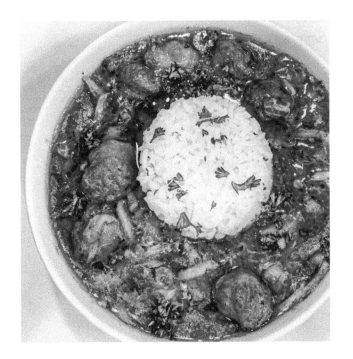

Directions:
1. In your slow cooker, mix sausages with chicken pieces, salt, pepper, bell peppers, oregano, onion, thyme, garlic powder, mustard powder, tomatoes, cayenne, chili and Creole seasoning.
2. Cover and cook on Low for 7 hours.
3. Uncover pot again, stir gumbo and divide into bowls.
4. Serve hot.
Enjoy!

Nutrition: calories 360, fat 23, fiber 2, carbs 6, protein 23

Tender Chicken Thighs

Preparation time: 10 minutes
Cooking time: 45 minutes
Servings: 4

Ingredients:
3 tablespoons ghee
8 ounces mushrooms, sliced
2 tablespoons gruyere cheese, grated
Salt and black pepper to the taste
2 garlic cloves, minced
6 chicken thighs, skin and bone-in

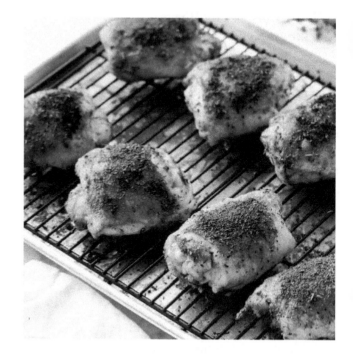

Directions:
1. Heat up a pan with 1 tablespoon ghee over medium heat, add chicken thighs, season with salt and pepper, cook for 3 minutes on each side and arrange them in a baking dish.
2. Heat up the pan again with the rest of the ghee over medium heat, add garlic, stir and cook for 1 minute.
3. Add mushrooms and stir well.
4. Add salt and pepper, stir and cook for 10 minutes.
5. Spoon these over chicken, sprinkle cheese, introduce in the oven at 350 degrees F and bake for 30 minutes.
6. Turn oven to broiler and broil everything for a couple more minutes.
7. Divide between plates and serve.
Enjoy!

Nutrition: calories 340, fat 31, fiber 3, carbs 5, protein 64

Tasty Crusted Chicken

Preparation time: 10 minutes
Cooking time: 20 minutes
Servings: 4

Ingredients:
1 egg, whisked
Salt and black pepper to the taste
3 tablespoons coconut oil
1 and ½ cups pecans, chopped
4 chicken breasts
Salt and black pepper to the taste

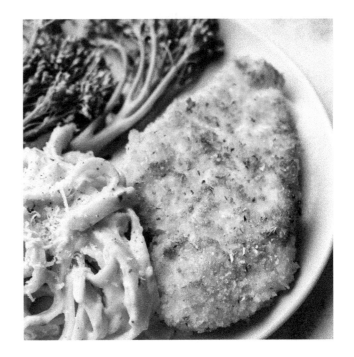

Directions:
1. Put pecans in a bowl and the whisked egg in another.
2. Season chicken, dip in egg and then in pecans.
3. Heat up a pan with the oil over medium high heat, add chicken and cook until it's brown on both sides.
4. Transfer chicken pieces to a baking sheet, introduce in the oven and bake at 350 degrees F for 10 minutes.
5. Divide between plates and serve.
Enjoy!

Nutrition: calories 320, fat 12, fiber 4, carbs 1, protein 30

Pepperoni Chicken Bake

Preparation time: 10 minutes
Cooking time: 55 minutes
Servings: 6

Ingredients:
14 ounces low carb pizza sauce
1 tablespoon coconut oil
4 medium chicken breasts, skinless and boneless
Salt and black pepper to the taste
1 teaspoon oregano, dried
6 ounces mozzarella, sliced
1 teaspoon garlic powder
2 ounces pepperoni, sliced

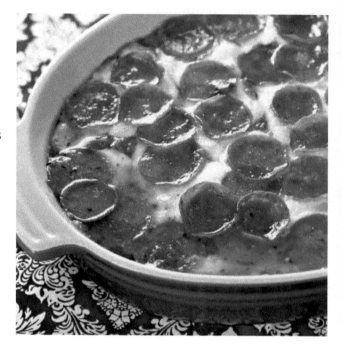

Directions:
1. Put pizza sauce in a small pot, bring to a boil over medium heat, simmer for 20 minutes and take off heat.
2. In a bowl, mix chicken with salt, pepper, garlic powder and oregano and stir.
3. Heat up a pan with the coconut oil over medium high heat, add chicken pieces, cook for 2 minutes on each side and transfer them to a baking dish.
4. Add mozzarella slices on top, spread sauce, top with pepperoni slices, introduce in the oven at 400 degrees F and bake for 30 minutes.
5. Divide between plates and serve.
Enjoy!

Nutrition: calories 320, fat 10, fiber 6, carbs 3, protein 27

Fried Chicken

Preparation time: 24 hours
Cooking time: 20 minutes
Servings: 4

Ingredients:
3 chicken breasts, cut into strips
4 ounces pork rinds, crushed
2 cups coconut oil
16 ounces jarred pickle juice
2 eggs, whisked

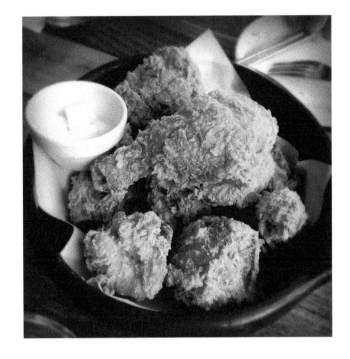

Directions:
1. In a bowl, mix chicken breast pieces with pickle juice, stir, cover and keep in the fridge for 24 hours.
2. Put eggs in a bowl and pork rinds in another one.
3. Dip chicken pieces in egg and then in rings and coat well.
4. Heat up a pan with the oil over medium high heat, add chicken pieces, fry them for 3 minutes on each side, transfer them to paper towels and drain grease.
5. Serve with a keto aioli sauce on the side.
Enjoy!

Nutrition: calories 260, fat 5, fiber 1, carbs 2, protein 20

Chicken Calzone

Preparation time: 10 minutes
Cooking time: 1 hour
Servings: 12

Ingredients:
2 eggs
1 keto pizza crust
½ cup parmesan, grated
1 pound chicken breasts, skinless, boneless and each sliced in halves
½ cup keto marinara sauce
1 teaspoon Italian seasoning
1 teaspoon onion powder
1 teaspoon garlic powder
Salt and black pepper to the taste
¼ cup flaxseed, ground
8 ounces provolone cheese

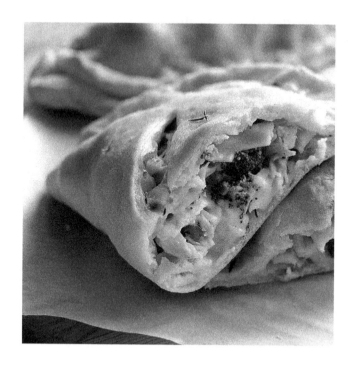

Directions:
1. In a bowl, mix Italian seasoning with onion powder, garlic powder, salt, pepper, flaxseed and parmesan and stir well.
2. In another bowl, mix eggs with a pinch of salt and pepper and whisk well.
3. Dip chicken pieces in eggs and then in seasoning mix, place all pieces on a lined baking sheet and bake in the oven at 350 degrees F for 30 minutes.
4. Put pizza crust dough on a lined baking sheet and spread half of the provolone cheese on half
5. Take chicken out of the oven, chop and spread over provolone cheese.
6. Add marinara sauce and then the rest of the cheese.
7. Cover all these with the other half of the dough and shape your calzone.
8. Seal its edges, introduce in the oven at 350 degrees F and bake for 20 minutes more.
9. Leave calzone to cool down before slicing and serving.
Enjoy!

Nutrition: calories 340, fat 8, fiber 2, carbs 6, protein 20

Mexican Chicken Soup

Preparation time: 10 minutes
Cooking time: 4 hours
Servings: 6

Ingredients:
1 and ½ pounds chicken tights, skinless,
boneless and cubed
15 ounces chicken stock
15 ounces canned chunky salsa
8 ounces Monterey jack

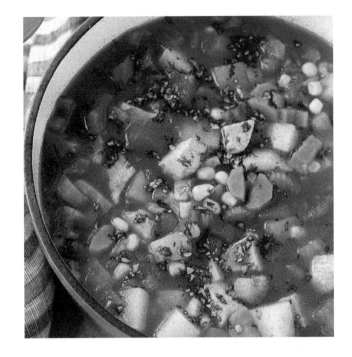

Directions:
1. In your slow cooker, mix chicken with stock, salsa and cheese, stir, cover and cook on High for 4 hours.
2. Uncover pot, stir soup, divide into bowls and serve.
Enjoy!

Nutrition: calories 400, fat 22, fiber 3, carbs 6, protein 38

Simple Chicken Stir Fry

Preparation time: 10 minutes
Cooking time: 12 minutes
Servings: 2

Ingredients:
2 chicken thighs, skinless, boneless cut into thin strips
1 tablespoon sesame oil
1 teaspoon red pepper flakes
1 teaspoon onion powder
1 tablespoon ginger, grated
¼ cup tamari sauce
½ teaspoon garlic powder
½ cup water
1 tablespoon stevia
½ teaspoon xanthan gum
½ cup scallions, chopped
2 cups broccoli florets

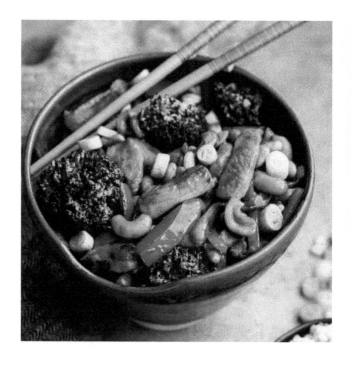

Directions:
1. Heat up a pan with the oil over medium high heat, add chicken and ginger, stir and cook for 3 minutes.
2. Add water, tamari sauce, onion powder, garlic powder, stevia, pepper flakes and xanthan gum, stir and cook for 5 minutes.
3. Add broccoli and scallions, stir, cook for 2 minutes more and divide between plates.
4. Serve hot.
Enjoy!

Nutrition: calories 210, fat 10, fiber 3, carbs 5, protein 20

Spinach And Artichoke Chicken

Preparation time: 10 minutes
Cooking time: 50 minutes
Servings: 4

Ingredients:
4 ounces cream cheese
4 chicken breasts
10 ounces canned artichoke hearts, chopped
10 ounces spinach
½ cup parmesan, grated
1 tablespoon dried onion
1 tablespoon garlic, dried
Salt and black pepper to the taste
4 ounces mozzarella, shredded

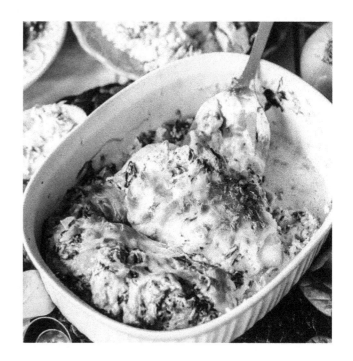

Directions:
1. Place chicken breasts on a lined baking sheet, season with salt and pepper, introduce in the oven at 400 degrees F and bake for 30 minutes.
2. In a bowl, mix artichokes with onion, cream cheese, parmesan, spinach, garlic, salt and pepper and stir.
3. Take chicken out of the oven, cut each piece in the middle,
divide artichokes mix, sprinkle mozzarella, introduce in the oven at 400 degrees F and bake for 15 minutes more.
4. Serve hot.
Enjoy!

Nutrition: calories 450, fat 23, fiber 1, carbs 3, protein 39

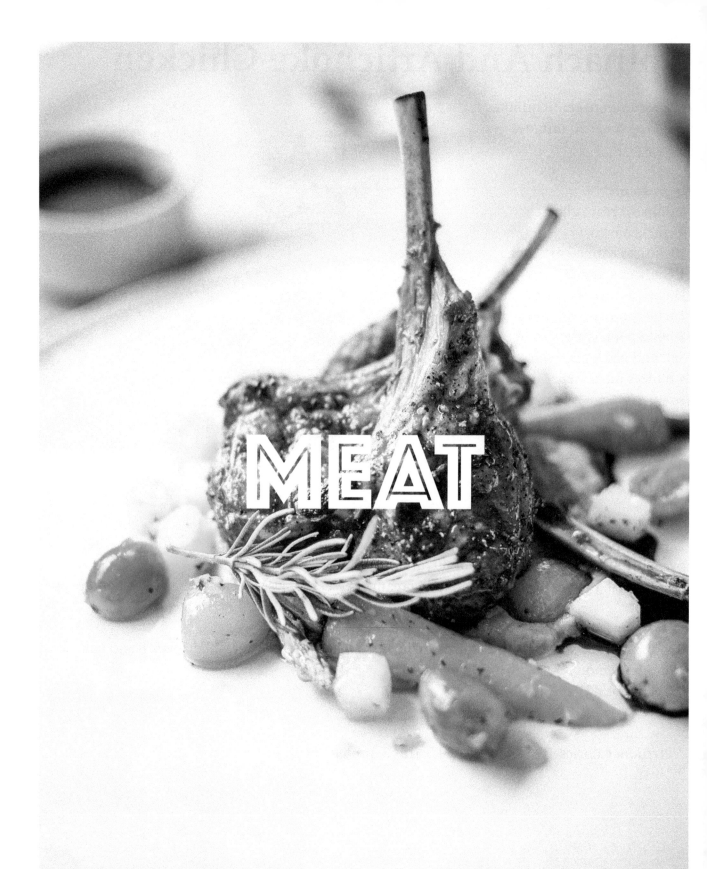

Tasty Roasted Pork Belly

Preparation time: 10 minutes
Cooking time: 1 hour and 30 minutes
Servings: 6

Ingredients:
2 tablespoons stevia
1 tablespoon lemon juice
1 quart water
17 ounces apples, cored and cut into wedges
2 pounds pork belly, scored
Salt and black pepper to the taste
A drizzle of olive oil

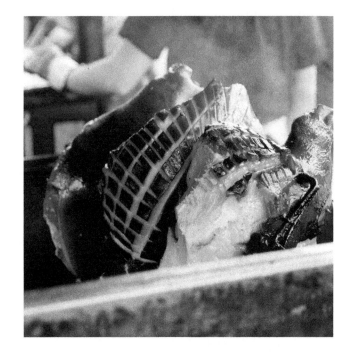

Directions:
1. In your blender, mix water with apples, lemon juice and stevia and pulse very well.
2. Put the pork belly in a steamer tray and steam for 1 hour.
3. Transfer pork belly to a baking sheet, rub with a drizzle of oil, season with salt and pepper and pour the apple sauce over it.
4. Introduce in the oven at 425 degrees F for 30 minutes.
5. Slice pork roast, divide between plates and serve with the applesauce on top.
Enjoy!

Nutrition: calories 456, fat 34, fiber 4, carbs 10, protein 25

Amazing Stuffed Pork

Preparation time: 10 minutes
Cooking time: 30 minutes
Servings: 4

Ingredients:
Zest of 2 limes
Zest from 1 orange
Juice from 1 orange
Juice from 2 limes
4 teaspoons garlic, minced
¾ cup olive oil
1 cup cilantro, chopped
1 cup mint, chopped
1 teaspoon oregano, dried
Salt and black pepper to the taste
2 teaspoons cumin, ground
4 pork loin steaks
2 pickles, chopped
4 ham slices
6 Swiss cheese slices
2 tablespoons mustard

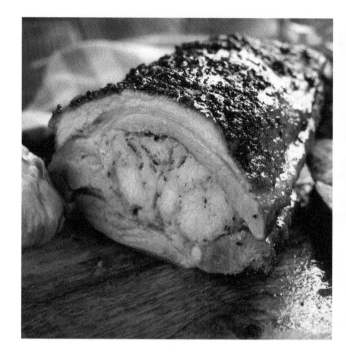

Directions:
1. In your food processor, mix lime zest and juice with orange zest and juice, garlic, oil, cilantro, mint, oregano, cumin, salt and pepper and blend well.
2. Season steaks with salt and pepper, place them into a bowl, add marinade you've made, toss to coat and leave aside for a couple of hours.
3. Place steaks on a working surface, divide pickles, cheese, mustard and ham on them, roll and secure with toothpicks.
4. Heat up a pan over medium high heat, add pork rolls, cook them for 2 minutes on each side and transfer them to a baking sheet.
5. Introduce in the oven at 350 degrees F and bake for 25 minutes.
6. Divide between plates and serve.
Enjoy!

Nutrition: calories 270, fat 7, fiber 2, carbs 3, protein 20

Delicious Pork Chops

Preparation time: 10 minutes
Cooking time: 40 minutes
Servings: 3

Ingredients:
8 ounces mushrooms, sliced
1 teaspoon garlic powder
1 yellow onion, chopped
1 cup mayonnaise
3 pork chops, boneless
1 teaspoon nutmeg
1 tablespoon balsamic vinegar
½ cup coconut oil

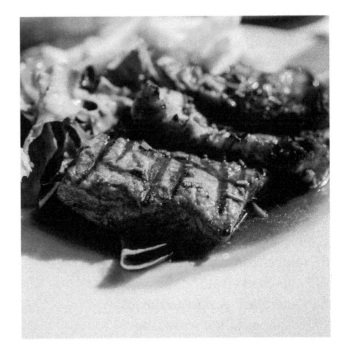

Directions:
1. Heat up a pan with the oil over medium heat, add mushrooms and onions, stir and cook for 4 minutes.
2. Add pork chops, season with nutmeg and garlic powder and brown on both sides.
3. Introduce pan in the oven at 350 degrees F and bake for 30 minutes.
4. Transfer pork chops to plates and keeps warm.
5. Heat up the pan over medium heat, add vinegar and mayo over mushrooms mix, stir well and take off heat.
6. Drizzle sauce over pork chops and serve.
Enjoy!

Nutrition: calories 600, fat 10, fiber 1, carbs 8, protein 30

Italian Pork Rolls

Preparation time: 10 minutes
Cooking time: 20 minutes
Servings: 6

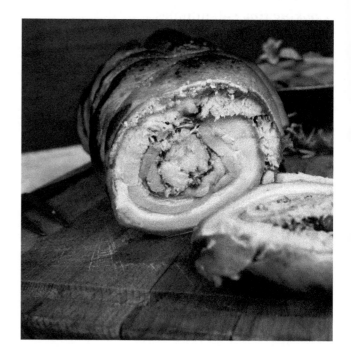

Ingredients:
6 prosciutto slices
2 tablespoons parsley, chopped
1 pound pork cutlets, thinly sliced
1/3 cup ricotta cheese
1 tablespoon coconut oil
¼ cup yellow onion, chopped
3 garlic cloves, minced
2 tablespoons parmesan, grated
15 ounces canned tomatoes, chopped
1/3 cup chicken stock
Salt and black pepper to the taste
½ teaspoon Italian seasoning

Directions:
1. Use a meat pounder to flatten pork pieces.
2. Place prosciutto slices on top of each piece, then divide ricotta, parsley and parmesan.
3. Roll each pork piece and secure with a toothpick.
4. Heat up a pan with the oil over medium heat, add pork rolls, cook until they are brown on both sides and transfer to a plate.
5. Heat up the pan again over medium heat, add garlic and onion, stir and cook for 5 minutes.
6. Add stock and cook for 3 minutes more.
7. Discard toothpicks from pork rolls and return them to the pan.
8. Add tomatoes, Italian seasoning, salt and pepper, stir, bring to a boil, reduce heat to medium-low, cover pan and cook for 30 minutes.
9. Divide between plates and serve.
Enjoy!

Nutrition: calories 280, fat 17, fiber 1, carbs 2, protein 34

Lemon And Garlic Pork

Preparation time: 10 minutes
Cooking time: 30 minutes
Servings: 4

Ingredients:
3 tablespoons ghee
4 pork steaks, bone in
1 cup chicken stock
Salt and black pepper to the taste
A pinch of lemon pepper
3 tablespoons coconut oil
6 garlic cloves, minced
2 tablespoons parsley, chopped
8 ounces mushrooms, roughly chopped
1 lemon, sliced

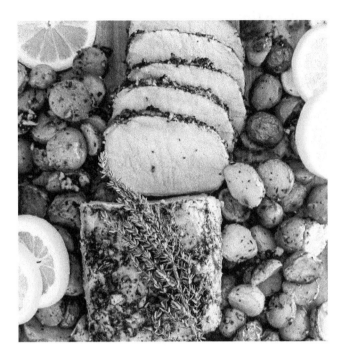

Directions:
1. Heat up a pan with 2 tablespoons ghee and 2 tablespoons oilover medium high heat, add pork steaks, season with salt and pepper, cook until they are brown on both sides and transfer to a plate.
2. Return pan to medium heat, add the rest of the ghee and oil and half of the stock.
3. Stir well and cook for 1 minute.
4. Add mushrooms and garlic, stir and cook for 4 minutes.
5. Add lemon slices, the rest of the stock, salt, pepper and lemon pepper, stir and cook everything for 5 minutes.
6. Return pork steaks to pan and cook everything for 10 minutes more.
7. Divide steaks and sauce between plates and serve.
Enjoy!

Nutrition: calories 456, fat 25, fiber 1, carbs 6, protein 40

Jamaican Pork

Preparation time: 10 minutes
Cooking time: 45 minutes
Servings: 12

Ingredients:
4 pounds pork shoulder
1 tablespoon coconut oil
½ cup beef stock
¼ cup Jamaican jerk spice mix

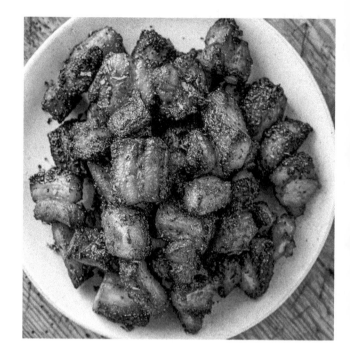

Directions:
1. Rub pork shoulder with Jamaican mix and place in your instant pot.
2. Add oil to the pot and set it to Sauté mode.
3. Add pork shoulder and brown it on all sides.
4. Add stock, cover pot and cook on High for 45 minutes.
5. Uncover pot, transfer pork to a platter, shred and serve.
Enjoy!

Nutrition: calories 267, fat 20, fiber 0, carbs 0, protein 24

Cranberry Pork Roast

Preparation time: 10 minutes
Cooking time: 8 hours
Servings: 4

Ingredients:
1 tablespoon coconut flour
Salt and black pepper to the taste
1 and ½ pounds pork loin
A pinch of mustard, ground
½ teaspoon ginger
2 tablespoons sukrin
2 tablespoons sukrin gold
½ cup cranberries
2 garlic cloves, minced
½ lemon sliced
¼ cup water

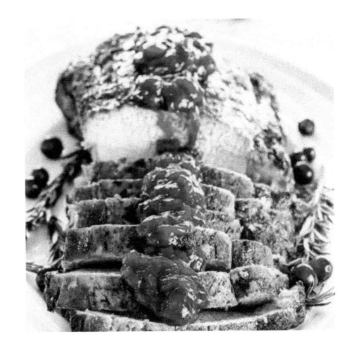

Directions:
1. In a bowl, mix ginger with mustard, salt, pepper and flour and stir.
2. Add roast, toss to coat and transfer meat to a Crockpot.
3. Add sukrin and sukrin gold, cranberries, garlic, water and lemon slices.
4. Cover pot and cook on Low for 8 hours.
5. Divide on plates, drizzle pan juices on top and serve.
Enjoy!

Nutrition: calories 430, fat 23, fiber 2, carbs 3, protein 45

Juicy Pork Chops

Preparation time: 10 minutes
Cooking time: 45 minutes
Servings: 4

Ingredients:
2 yellow onions, chopped
6 bacon slices, chopped
½ cup chicken stock
Salt and black pepper to the taste
4 pork chops

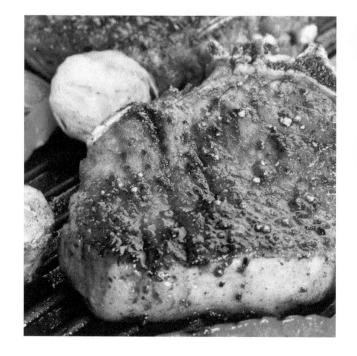

Directions:
1. Heat up a pan over medium heat, add bacon, stir, cook until it's crispy and transfer to a bowl.
2. Return pan to medium heat, add onions, some salt and pepper, stir, cover, cook for 15 minutes and transfer to the same bowl with the bacon.
3. Return pan once again to heat, increase to medium high, add pork chops, season with salt and pepper, brown for 3 minutes on one side, flip, reduce heat to medium and cook for 7 minutes more.
4. Add stock, stir and cook for 2 minutes more.
5. Return bacon and onions to the pan, stir, cook for 1 minute more, divide between plates and serve.
Enjoy!

Nutrition: calories 325, fat 18, fiber 1, carbs 6, protein 36

Simple And Fast Pork Chops

Preparation time: 10 minutes
Cooking time: 15 minutes
Servings: 4

Ingredients:
4 medium pork loin chops
1 teaspoon Dijon mustard
1 tablespoon Worcestershire sauce
1 teaspoon lemon juice
1 tablespoon water
Salt and black pepper to the taste
1 teaspoon lemon pepper
1 tablespoon ghee
1 tablespoon chives, chopped

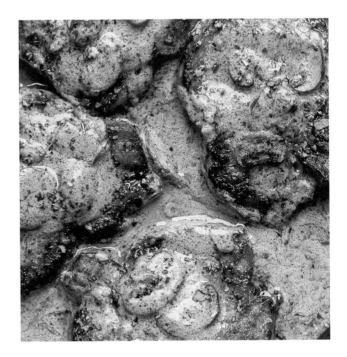

Directions:
1. In a bowl, mix water with Worcestershire sauce, mustard and lemon juice and whisk well.
2. Heat up a pan with the ghee over medium heat, add pork chops, season with salt, pepper and lemon pepper, cook them for 6 minutes, flip and cook for 6 more minutes.
3. Transfer pork chops to a platter and keep them warm for now.
4. Heat up the pan again, pour mustard sauce you've made and bring to a gentle simmer.
5. Pour this over pork, sprinkle chives and serve.
Enjoy!

Nutrition: calories 132, fat 5, fiber 1, carbs 1, protein 18

Mediterranean Pork

Preparation time: 10 minutes
Cooking time: 35 minutes
Servings: 4

Ingredients:
4 pork chops, bone-in
Salt and black pepper to the taste
1 teaspoon rosemary, dried
3 garlic cloves, minced

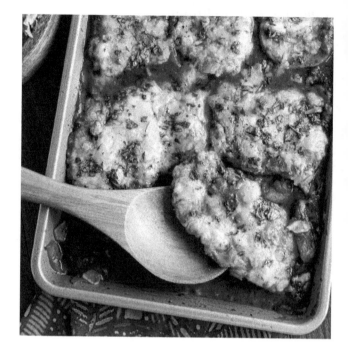

Directions:
1. Season pork chops with salt and pepper and place in a roasting pan.
2. Add rosemary and garlic, introduce in the oven at 425 degrees F and bake for 10 minutes.
3. Reduce heat to 350 degrees F and roast for 25 minutes more.
4. Slice pork, divide between plates and drizzle pan juices all over.
Enjoy!

Nutrition: calories 165, fat 2, fiber 1, carbs 2, protein 26

Simple Pork Chops Delight

Preparation time: 10 minutes
Cooking time: 40 minutes
Servings: 4

Ingredients:
4 pork chops
1 tablespoon oregano, chopped
2 garlic cloves, minced
1 tablespoon canola oil
15 ounces canned tomatoes, chopped
1 tablespoon tomato paste
Salt and black pepper to the taste
¼ cup tomato juice

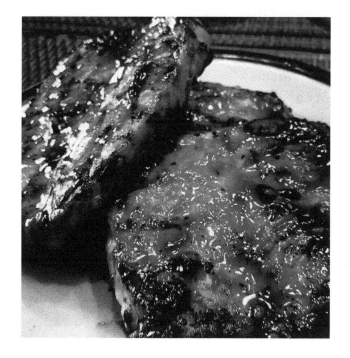

Directions:
1. Heat up a pan with the oil over medium high heat, add pork chops, season with salt and pepper, cook for 3 minutes, flip, cook for 3 minutes more and transfer to a plate.
2. Return pan to medium heat, add garlic, stir and cook for 10 seconds.
3. Add tomato juice, tomatoes and tomato paste, stir, bring to a boil and reduce heat to medium-low.
4. Add pork chops, stir, cover pan and simmer everything for 30 minutes.
5. Transfer pork chops to plates, add oregano to the pan, stir and cook for 2 minutes more.
6. Pour this over pork and serve.
Enjoy!

Nutrition: calories 210, fat 10, fiber 2, carbs 6, protein 19

Spicy Pork Chops

Preparation time: 4 hours and 10 minutes
Cooking time: 15 minutes
Servings: 4

Ingredients:
¼ cup lime juice
4 pork rib chops
1 tablespoon coconut oil, melted
2 garlic cloves, minced
1 tablespoon chili powder
1 teaspoon cinnamon, ground
2 teaspoons cumin, ground
Salt and black pepper to the taste
½ teaspoon hot pepper sauce
Sliced mango for serving

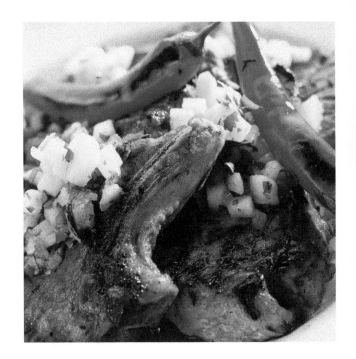

Directions:
1. In a bowl, mix lime juice with oil, garlic, cumin, cinnamon, chili powder, salt, pepper and hot pepper sauce and whisk well.
2. Add pork chops, toss to coat and leave aside in the fridge for 4 hours.
3. Place pork on preheated grill over medium heat, cook for 7 minutes, flip and cook for 7 minutes more.
4. Divide between plates and serve with mango slices on the side.
Enjoy!

Nutrition: calories 200, fat 8, fiber 1, carbs 3, protein 26

Tasty Thai Beef

Preparation time: 10 minutes
Cooking time: 10 minutes
Servings: 6

Ingredients:
1 cup beef stock
4 tablespoons peanut butter
¼ teaspoon garlic powder
¼ teaspoon onion powder
1 tablespoon coconut aminos
1 and ½ teaspoons lemon pepper
1 pound beef steak, cut into strips
Salt and black pepper to the taste
1 green bell pepper, chopped
3 green onions, chopped

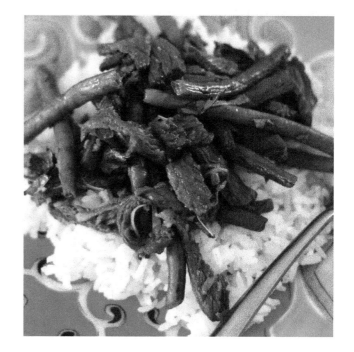

Directions:
1. In a bowl, mix peanut butter with stock, aminos and lemon pepper, stir well and leave aside.
2. Heat up a pan over medium high heat, add beef, season with salt, pepper, onion and garlic powder and cook for 7 minutes.
3. Add green pepper, stir and cook for 3 minutes more.
4. Add peanut sauce you've made at the beginning and green onions, stir, cook for 1 minute more, divide between plates and
serve.
Enjoy!

Nutrition: calories 224, fat 15, fiber 1, carbs 3, protein 19

The Best Beef Patties

Preparation time: 10 minutes
Cooking time: 35 minutes
Servings: 6

Ingredients:
½ cup bread crumbs
1 egg
Salt and black pepper to the taste
1 and ½ pounds beef, ground
10 ounces canned onion soup
1 tablespoon coconut flour
¼ cup ketchup
3 teaspoons Worcestershire sauce
½ teaspoon mustard powder
¼ cup water

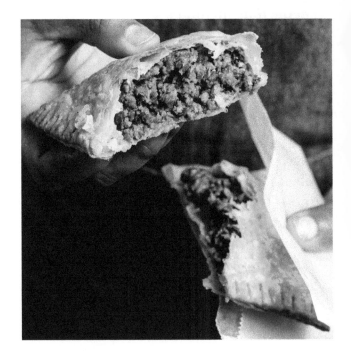

Directions:
1. In a bowl, mix 1/3 cup onion soup with beef, salt, pepper, egg and bread crumbs and stir well.
2. Heat up a pan over medium high heat, shape 6 patties from the beef mix, place them into the pan and brown on both sides.
3. Meanwhile, in a bowl, mix the rest of the soup with coconut flour, water, mustard powder, Worcestershire sauce and ketchup and stir well.
4. Pour this over beef patties, cover pan and cook for 20 minutes stirring from time to time.
5. Divide between plates and serve.
Enjoy!

Nutrition: calories 332, fat 18, fiber 1, carbs 7, protein 25

Amazing Beef Roast

Preparation time: 10 minutes
Cooking time: 1 hour and 15 minutes
Servings: 4

Ingredients:
3 and ½ pounds beef roast
4 ounces mushrooms, sliced
12 ounces beef stock
1 ounce onion soup mix
½ cup Italian dressing

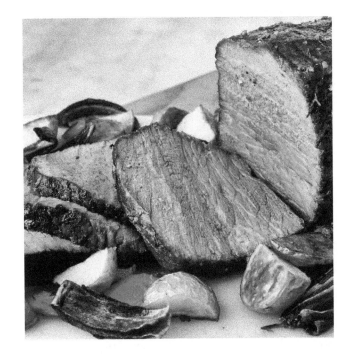

Directions:
1. In a bowl, mix stock with onion soup mix and Italian dressing and stir.
2. Put beef roast in a pan, add mushrooms, stock mix, cover with tin foil, introduce in the oven at 300 degrees F and bake for 1
hour and 15 minutes.
3. Leave roast to cool down a bit, slice and serve with the gravy on top.
Enjoy!

Nutrition: calories 700, fat 56, fiber 2, carbs 10, protein 70

Beef Zucchini Cups

Preparation time: 10 minutes
Cooking time: 35 minutes
Servings: 4

Ingredients:
2 garlic cloves, minced
1 teaspoon cumin, ground
1 tablespoon coconut oil
1 pound beef, ground
½ cup red onion, chopped
1 teaspoon smoked paprika
Salt and black pepper to the taste
3 zucchinis, sliced in halves lengthwise
and insides scooped out
¼ cup cilantro, chopped
½ cup cheddar cheese, shredded
1 and ½ cups keto enchilada sauce
Some chopped avocado for serving
Some green onions, chopped for serving
Some tomatoes, chopped for serving

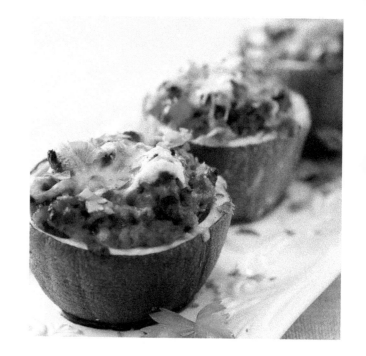

Directions:
1. Heat up a pan with the oil over medium high heat, add red onions, stir and cook for 2 minutes.
2. Add beef, stir and brown for a couple of minutes.
3. Add paprika, salt, pepper, cumin and garlic, stir and cook for 2 minutes.
4. Place zucchini halves in a baking pan, stuff each with beef, pour enchilada sauce on top and sprinkle cheddar cheese.
5. Bake covered in the oven at 350 degrees F for 20 minutes.
6. Uncover the pan, sprinkle cilantro and bake for 5 minutes more.
7. Sprinkle avocado, green onions and tomatoes on top, divide between plates and serve.
Enjoy!

Nutrition: calories 222, fat 10, fiber 2, carbs 8, protein 21

Beef Meatballs Casserole

Preparation time: 10 minutes
Cooking time: 50 minutes
Servings: 8

Ingredients:
1/3 cup almond flours
2 eggs
1 pound beef sausage, chopped
1 pound ground beef
Salt and black pepper to taste
1 tablespoons parsley, dried
¼ teaspoon red pepper flakes
¼ cup parmesan, grated
¼ teaspoon onion powder
½ teaspoon garlic powder
¼ teaspoon oregano, dried
1 cup ricotta cheese
2 cups keto marinara sauce
1 and ½ cups mozzarella cheese, shredded

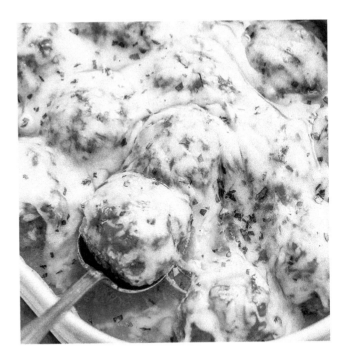

Directions:
1. In a bowl, mix sausage with beef, salt, pepper, almond flour, parsley, pepper flakes, onion powder, garlic powder, oregano, parmesan and eggs and stir well.
2. Shape meatballs, place them on a lined baking sheet, introduce in the oven at 375 degrees F and bake for 15 minutes.
3. Take meatballs out of the oven, transfer them to a baking dish and cover with half of the marinara sauce.
4. Add ricotta cheese all over, then pour the rest of the marinara sauce.
5. Sprinkle mozzarella all over, introduce dish in the oven at 375 degrees F and bake for 30 minutes.
6. Leave your meatballs casserole to cool down a bit before cutting and serving.
Enjoy!

Nutrition: calories 456, fat 35, fiber 3, carbs 4, protein 32

Beef And Tomato Stuffed Squash

Preparation time: 10 minutes
Cooking time: 1 hour
Servings: 2

Ingredients:
2 pounds spaghetti squash, pricked with a fork
Salt and black pepper to the taste
3 garlic cloves, minced
1 yellow onion, chopped
1 Portobello mushroom, sliced
28 ounces canned tomatoes, chopped
1 teaspoon oregano, dried
¼ teaspoon cayenne pepper
½ teaspoon thyme, dried
1 pound beef, ground
1 green bell pepper, chopped

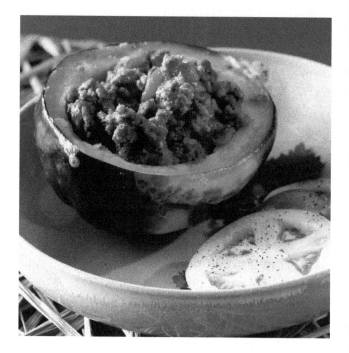

Directions:
1. Place spaghetti squash on a lined baking sheet, introduce in the oven at 400 degrees F and bake for 40 minutes.
2. Cut in half, leave aside to cool down, remove seeds and leave aside.
3. Heat up a pan over medium high heat, add meat, garlic, onion and mushroom, stir and cook until meat browns.
4. Add salt, pepper, thyme, oregano, cayenne, tomatoes and green pepper, stir and cook for 10 minutes.
5. Stuff squash halves with this beef mix, introduce in the oven at 400 degrees F and bake for 10 minutes.
6. Divide between 2 plates and serve.
Enjoy!

Nutrition: calories 260, fat 7, fiber 2, carbs 4, protein 10

Tasty Beef Chili

Preparation time: 10 minutes
Cooking time: 8 hours
Servings: 4

Ingredients:
1 red onion, chopped
2 and ½ pounds beef, ground
15 ounces canned tomatoes and green chilies, chopped
6 ounces tomato paste
½ cup pickled jalapenos, chopped
4 tablespoons garlic, minced
3 celery ribs, chopped
2 tablespoons coconut aminos
4 tablespoons chili powder
Salt and black pepper to the taste
A pinch of cayenne pepper
2 tablespoons cumin, ground
1 teaspoon onion powder
1 teaspoon garlic powder
1 bay leaf
1 teaspoon oregano, dried

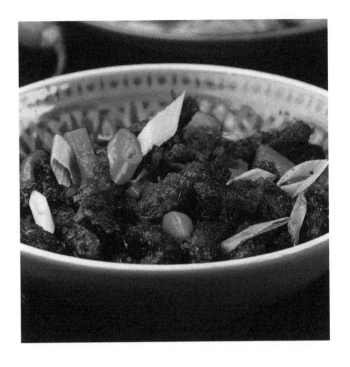

Directions:
1. Heat up a pan over medium high heat, add half of the onion, beef, half of the garlic, salt and pepper, stir and cook until meat browns.
2. Transfer this to your slow cooker, add the rest of the onion and garlic, but also, jalapenos, celery, tomatoes and chilies, tomato paste, canned tomatoes, coconut aminos, chili powder, salt, pepper, cumin, garlic powder, onion powder, oregano and bay leaf, stir, cover and cook on Low for 8 hours.
3. Divide into bowls and serve.
Enjoy!

Nutrition: calories 137, fat 6, fiber 2, carbs 5, protein 17

Glazed Beef Meatloaf

Preparation time: 10 minutes
Cooking time: 1 hour and 10 minutes
Servings: 6

Ingredients:
1 cup white mushrooms, chopped
3 pounds beef, ground
2 tablespoons parsley, chopped
2 garlic cloves, minced
½ cup yellow onion, chopped
¼ cup red bell pepper, chopped
½ cup almond flour
1/3 cup parmesan, grated
3 eggs
Salt and black pepper to the taste
1 teaspoon balsamic vinegar
For the glaze:
1 tablespoon swerve
2 tablespoons sugar-free ketchup
2 cups balsamic vinegar

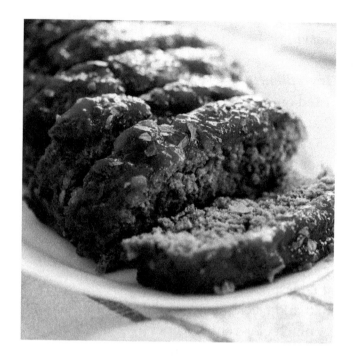

Directions:
1. In a bowl, mix beef with salt, pepper, mushrooms, garlic, onion, bell pepper, parsley, almond flour, parmesan, 1 teaspoon vinegar, salt, pepper and eggs and stir very well.
2. Transfer this into a loaf pan and bake in the oven at 375 degrees F for 30 minutes.
3. Meanwhile, heat up a small pan over medium heat, add ketchup, swerve and 2 cups vinegar, stir well and cook for 20 minutes.
4. Take meatloaf out of the oven, spread the glaze over, introduce in the oven at the same temperature and bake for 20 minutes more.
5. Leave meatloaf to cool down, slice and serve it.
Enjoy!

Nutrition: calories 264, fat 14, fiber 3, carbs 5, protein 24

Delicious Beef And Tzatziki

Preparation time: 10 minutes
Cooking time: 15 minutes
Servings: 6

Ingredients:
¼ cup almond milk
17 ounces beef, ground
1 yellow onion, grated
5 bread slices, torn
1 egg, whisked
¼ cup parsley, chopped
Salt and black pepper to the taste
2 garlic cloves, minced
¼ cup mint, chopped
2 and ½ teaspoons oregano, dried
¼ cup olive oil
7 ounces cherry tomatoes, cut in halves
1 cucumber, thinly sliced
1 cup baby spinach
1 and ½ tablespoons lemon juice
7 ounces jarred tzatziki

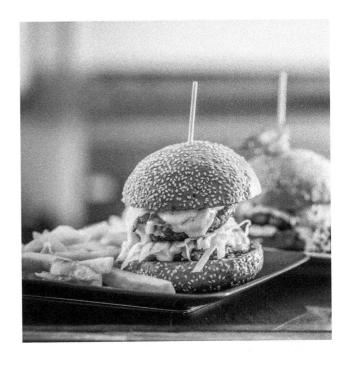

Directions:
1. Put torn bread in a bowl, add milk and leave aside for 3 minutes.
2. Squeeze bread, chop and put into a bowl.
3. Add beef, egg, salt, pepper, oregano, mint, parsley, garlic and onion and stir well.
4. Shape balls from this mix and place on a working surface.
5. Heat up a pan with half of the oil over medium high heat, add meatballs, cook them for 8 minutes flipping them from time to time and transfer them all to a tray.
6. In a salad bowl, mix spinach with cucumber and tomato.
7. Add meatballs, the rest of the oil, some salt, pepper and lemon juice.
8. Also add tzatziki, toss to coat and serve.
Enjoy!

Nutrition: calories 200, fat 4, fiber 1, carbs 3, protein 7

Meatballs And Tasty Mushroom Sauce

Preparation time: 10 minutes
Cooking time: 25 minutes
Servings: 6

Ingredients:
2 pounds beef, ground
Salt and black pepper to the taste
½ teaspoon garlic powder
1 tablespoon coconut aminos
¼ cup beef stock
¾ cup almond flour
1 tablespoon parsley, chopped
1 tablespoon onion flakes
For the sauce:
1 cup yellow onion, chopped
2 cups mushrooms, sliced
2 tablespoons bacon fat
2 tablespoons ghee
½ teaspoon coconut aminos
¼ cup sour cream
½ cup beef stock
Salt and black pepper to the taste

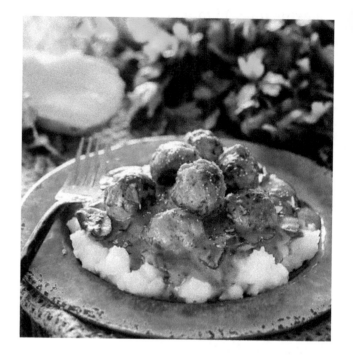

Directions:
1. In a bowl, mix beef with salt, pepper, garlic powder, 1 tablespoons coconut aminos, ¼ cup beef stock, almond flour, parsley and onion flakes, stir well, shape 6 patties, place them on a baking sheet, introduce in the oven at 375 degrees F and bake for 18 minutes.
2. Meanwhile, heat up a pan with the ghee and the bacon fat over medium heat, add mushrooms, stir and cook for 4 minutes.
3. Add onions, stir and cook for 4 minutes more.
4. Add ½ teaspoon coconut aminos, sour cream and ½ cup beef stock, stir well and bring to a simmer.
5. Take off heat, add salt and pepper and stir well.
6. Divide beef patties between plates and serve with mushroom sauce on top.
Enjoy!

Nutrition: calories 435, fat 23, fiber 4, carbs 6, protein 32

Beef And Sauerkraut Soup

Preparation time: 10 minutes
Cooking time: 1 hour and 20 minutes
Servings: 8

Ingredients:
3 teaspoons olive oil
1 pound beef, ground
14 ounces beef stock
2 cups chicken stock
14 ounces canned tomatoes and juice
1 tablespoon stevia
14 ounces sauerkraut, chopped
1 tablespoon gluten free Worcestershire sauce
4 bay leaves
Salt and black pepper to the taste
3 tablespoons parsley, chopped
1 onion, chopped
1 teaspoon sage, dried
1 tablespoon garlic, minced
2 cups water

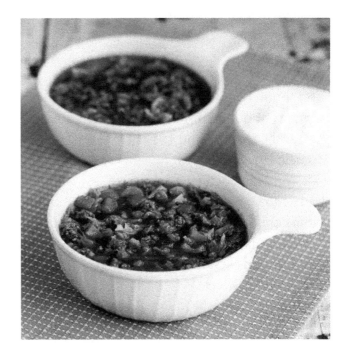

Directions:
1. Heat up a pan with 1 teaspoon oil over medium heat, add beef, stir and brown for 10 minutes.
2. Meanwhile, in a pot, mix chicken and beef stock with sauerkraut, stevia, canned tomatoes, Worcestershire sauce, parsley, sage and bay leaves, stir and bring to a simmer over medium heat.
3. Add beef to soup, stir and continue simmering.
4. Heat up the same pan with the rest of the oil over medium heat, add onions, stir and cook for 2 minutes. Add garlic, stir, cook for 1 minute more and add this to the soup.
5. Reduce heat to soup and simmer it for 1 hour.
6. Add salt, pepper and water, stir and cook for 15 minutes more.
7. Divide into bowls and serve.
Enjoy!

Nutrition: calories 250, fat 5, fiber 1, carbs 3, protein 12

Ground Beef Casserole

Preparation time: 10 minutes
Cooking time: 35 minutes
Servings: 6

Ingredients:
2 teaspoons onion flakes
1 tablespoon gluten free Worcestershire sauce
2 pounds beef, ground
2 garlic cloves, minced
Salt and black pepper to the taste
1 cup mozzarella cheese, shredded
2 cups cheddar cheese, shredded
1 cup Russian dressing
2 tablespoons sesame seeds, toasted
20 dill pickle slices
1 romaine lettuce head, torn

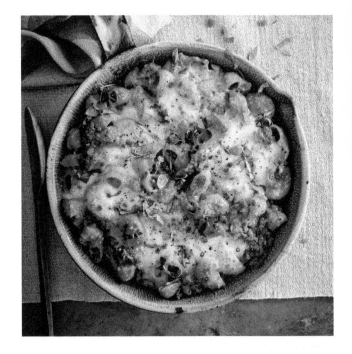

Directions:
1. Heat up a pan over medium heat, add beef, onion flakes, Worcestershire sauce, salt, pepper and garlic, stir and cook for
5 minutes.
2. Transfer this to a baking dish, add 1 cup cheddar cheese over it and also the mozzarella and half of the Russian dressing.
3. Stir and spread evenly.
4. Arrange pickle slices on top, sprinkle the rest of the cheddar and the sesame seeds, introduce in the oven at 350 degrees f and bake for 20 minutes.
5. Turn oven to broil and broil the casserole for 5 minutes more.
6. Divide lettuce on plates, top with a beef casserole and the rest of the Russian dressing.
Enjoy!

Nutrition: calories 554, fat 51, fiber 3, carbs 5, protein 45

Delicious Zoodles And Beef

Preparation time: 10 minutes
Cooking time: 20 minutes
Servings: 5

Ingredients:
1 pound beef, ground
1 yellow onion, chopped
2 garlic cloves, minced
14 ounces canned tomatoes, chopped
1 tablespoon rosemary, dried
1 tablespoon sage, dried
1 tablespoon oregano, dried
1 tablespoon basil, dried
1 tablespoon marjoram, dried
Salt and black pepper to the taste
2 zucchinis, cut with a spiralizer

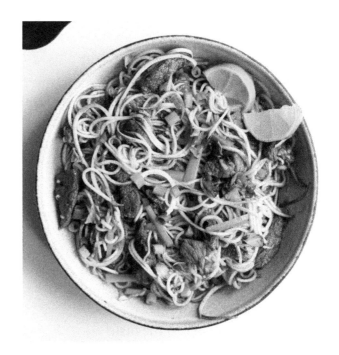

Directions:
1. Heat up a pan over medium heat, add garlic and onion, stir and brown for a couple of minutes.
2. Add beef, stir and cook for 6 minutes more.
3. Add tomatoes, salt, pepper, rosemary, sage, oregano, marjoram and basil, stir and simmer for 15 minutes.
4. Divide zoodles into bowls, add beef mix and serve.
Enjoy!

Nutrition: calories 320, fat 13, fiber 4, carbs 12, protein 40

Jamaican Beef Pies

Preparation time: 10 minutes
Cooking time: 35 minutes
Servings: 12

Ingredients:
3 garlic cloves, minced, ½ pound beef, ground
½ pound pork, ground, ½ cup water
1 small onion, chopped
2 habanero peppers, chopped
1 teaspoon Jamaican curry powder
1 teaspoon thyme, dried
2 teaspoons coriander, ground,
½ teaspoon allspice
2 teaspoons cumin, ground,
½ teaspoon turmeric
A pinch of cloves, ground
Salt and black pepper to the taste
1 teaspoon garlic powder, ¼ teaspoon stevia powder
2 tablespoons ghee, For the crust:
4 tablespoons ghee, melted, 6 ounces cream cheese
A pinch of salt, 1 teaspoon turmeric, ¼ teaspoon stevia, ½ teaspoon baking powder
1 and ½ cups flax meal, 2 tablespoons water, ½ cup coconut flour

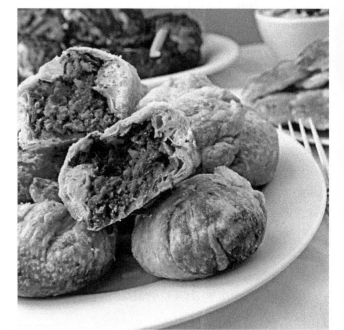

Directions:
1. In your blender, mix onion with habaneros, garlic and ½ cup water.
2. Heat up a pan over medium heat, add pork and beef meat, stir and cook for 3 minutes.
3. Add onions mix, stir and cook for 2 minutes more. Add garlic, onion, curry powder, ½ teaspoon turmeric, thyme, coriander, cumin, allspice, cloves, salt, pepper, stevia powder and garlic powder, stir well and cook for 3 minutes. Add 2 tablespoons ghee, stir until it melts and take this off heat. Meanwhile, in a bowl, mix 1 teaspoon turmeric, with ¼ teaspoon stevia, baking powder, flax meal and coconut flour and stir. In a separate bowl, mix 4 tablespoons ghee with 2 tablespoons water and cream cheese and stir. Combine the 2 mixtures and mix until you obtain a dough. Shape 12 balls from this mix, place them on a parchment paper and roll each into a circle.
4. Divide beef and pork mix on one half of the dough circles, cover with the other halves, seal edges and arrange them all on a lined baking sheet.
5. Bake your pies in the oven at 350 degrees F for 25 minutes. Serve them warm. Enjoy!

Nutrition: calories 267, fat 23, fiber 1, carbs 3, protein 12

Amazing Goulash

Preparation time: 10 minutes
Cooking time: 20 minutes
Servings: 5

Ingredients:
2 ounces bell pepper, chopped
1 and ½ pounds beef, ground
Salt and black pepper to the taste
2 cups cauliflower florets
¼ cup onion, chopped
14 ounces canned tomatoes and their juice
¼ teaspoon garlic powder
1 tablespoon tomato paste
14 ounces water

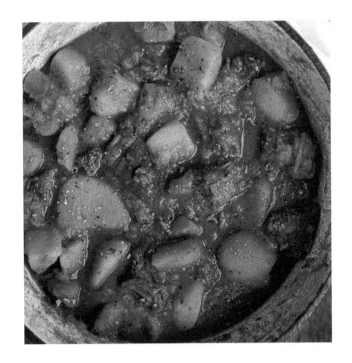

Directions:
1. Heat up a pan over medium heat, add beef, stir and brown for 5 minutes.
2. Add onion and bell pepper, stir and cook for 4 minutes more.
3. Add cauliflower, tomatoes and their juice and water, stir, bring to a simmer, cover pan and cook for 5 minutes.
4. Add tomato paste, garlic powder, salt and pepper, stir, take off heat, divide into bowls and serve.
Enjoy!

Nutrition: calories 275, fat 7, fiber 2, carbs 4, protein 10

Beef And Eggplant Casserole

Preparation time: 30 minutes
Cooking time: 4 hours
Servings: 12

Ingredients:
1 tablespoon olive oil
2 pounds beef, ground
2 cups eggplant, chopped
Salt and black pepper to the taste
2 teaspoons mustard
2 teaspoons gluten free Worcestershire sauce
28 ounces canned tomatoes, chopped
2 cups mozzarella, grated
16 ounces tomato sauce
2 tablespoons parsley, chopped
1 teaspoon oregano, dried

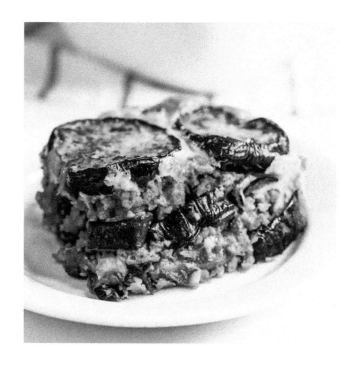

Directions:
1. Season eggplant pieces with salt and pepper, leave them aside for 30 minutes, squeeze water a bit, put them into a bowl, add the olive oil and toss them to coat.
2. In another bowl, mix beef with salt, pepper, mustard and Worcestershire sauce and stir well.
3. Press them on the bottom of a crock pot.
4. Add eggplant and spread.
5. Also add tomatoes, tomato sauce, parsley, oregano and mozzarella.
6. Cover Crockpot and cook on Low for 4 hours.
7. Divide casserole between plates and serve hot.
Enjoy!

Nutrition: calories 200, fat 12, fiber 2, carbs 6, protein 15

Braised Lamb Chops

Preparation time: 10 minutes
Cooking time: 2 hours and 20 minutes
Servings: 4

Ingredients:
8 lamb chops
1 teaspoon garlic powder
Salt and black pepper to the taste
2 teaspoons mint, crushed
A drizzle of olive oil
1 shallot, chopped, 1 cup white wine
Juice of ½ lemon, 1 bay leaf
2 cups beef stock
Some chopped parsley for serving
For the sauce:, 2 cups cranberries
½ teaspoon rosemary, chopped
½ cup swerve, 1 teaspoon mint, dried
Juice of ½ lemon, 1 teaspoon ginger, grated
1 cup water, 1 teaspoon harissa paste

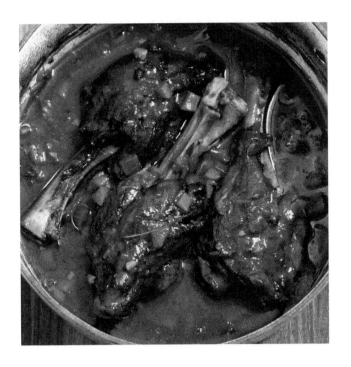

Directions:
1. In a bowl, mix lamb chops with salt, pepper, 1 teaspoon garlic powder and 2 teaspoons mint and rub well.
2. Heat up a pan with a drizzle of oil over medium high heat, add lamb chops, brown them on all sides and transfer to a plate.
3. Heat up the same pan again over medium high heat, add shallots, stir and cook for 1 minute.
4. Add wine and bay leaf, stir and cook for 4 minutes.
5. Add 2 cups beef stock, parsley and juice from ½ lemon, stir and simmer for 5 minutes.
6. Return lamb, stir and cook for 10 minutes.
7. Cover pan and introduce it in the oven at 350 degrees F for 2 hours.
8. Meanwhile, heat up a pan over medium high heat, add cranberries, swerve, rosemary, 1 teaspoon mint, juice from ½ lemon, ginger, water and harissa paste, stir, bring to a simmer for 15 minutes.
9. Take lamb chops out of the oven, divide them between plates, drizzle the cranberry sauce over them and serve.

Nutrition: calories 450, fat 34, fiber 2, carbs 6, protein 26

Amazing Lamb Salad

Preparation time: 10 minutes
Cooking time: 35 minutes
Servings: 4

Ingredients:
1 tablespoon olive oil
3 pounds leg of lamb, bone discarded
and butterflied
Salt and black pepper to the taste
1 teaspoon cumin, ground
A pinch of thyme, dried
2 garlic cloves, minced
For the salad:
4 ounces feta cheese, crumbled
½ cup pecans
2 cups spinach
1 and ½ tablespoons lemon juice
¼ cup olive oil
1 cup mint, chopped

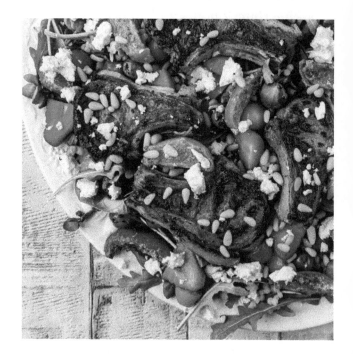

Directions:
1. Rub lamb with salt, pepper, 1 tablespoon oil, thyme, cumin and minced garlic, place on pre-heated grill over medium high heat and cook for 40 minutes, flipping once.
2. Meanwhile, spread pecans on a lined baking sheet, introduce in the oven at 350 degrees F and toast for 10 minutes.
3. Transfer grilled lamb to a cutting board, leave aside to cool down and slice.
4. In a salad bowl, mix spinach with 1 cup mint, feta cheese, ¼ cup olive oil, lemon juice, toasted pecans, salt and pepper and toss to coat.
5. Add lamb slices on top and serve.
Enjoy!

Nutrition: calories 334, fat 33, fiber 3, carbs 5, protein 7

Moroccan Lamb

Preparation time: 10 minutes
Cooking time: 15 minutes
Servings: 4

Ingredients:
2 teaspoons paprika
2 garlic cloves, minced
2 teaspoons oregano, dried
2 tablespoons sumac
12 lamb cutlets
¼ cup olive oil
2 tablespoons water
2 teaspoons cumin, ground
4 carrots, sliced
¼ cup parsley, chopped
2 teaspoons harissa
1 tablespoon red wine vinegar
Salt and black pepper to the taste
2 tablespoons black olives, pitted and sliced
6 radishes, thinly sliced

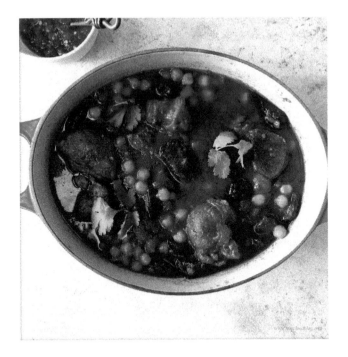

Directions:
1. In a bowl, mix cutlets with paprika, garlic, oregano, sumac, salt, pepper, half of the oil and the water and rub well.
2. Put carrots in a pot, add water to cover, bring to a boil over medium high heat, cook for 2 minutes drain and put them in a salad bowl.
3. Add olives and radishes over carrots.
4. In another bowl, mix harissa with the rest of the oil, parsley, cumin, vinegar and a splash of water and stir well.
5. Add this to carrots mix, season with salt and pepper and toss to coat.
6. Heat up a kitchen grill over medium high heat, add lamb cutlets, grill them for 3 minutes on each side and divide them between plates.
7. Add carrots salad on the side and serve.
Enjoy!

Nutrition: calories 245, fat 32, fiber 6, carbs 4, protein 34

Delicious Lamb And Mustard Sauce

Preparation time: 10 minutes
Cooking time: 20 minutes
Servings: 4

Ingredients:
2 tablespoons olive oil
1 tablespoon fresh rosemary, chopped
2 garlic cloves, minced
1 and ½ pounds lamb chops
Salt and black pepper to the taste
1 tablespoon shallot, chopped
2/3 cup heavy cream
½ cup beef stock
1 tablespoon mustard
2 teaspoons gluten free Worcestershire sauce
2 teaspoons lemon juice
1 teaspoon erythritol
2 tablespoons ghee
A spring of rosemary
A spring of thyme

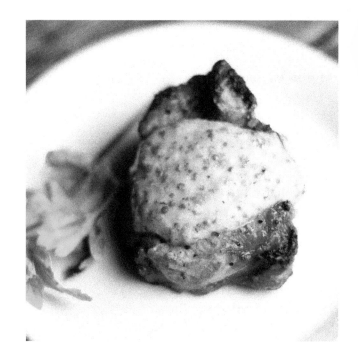

Directions:
1. In a bowl, mix 1 tablespoon oil with garlic, salt, pepper and rosemary and whisk well.
2. Add lamb chops, toss to coat and leave aside for a few minutes.
3. Heat up a pan with the rest of the oil over medium high heat, add lamb chops, reduce heat to medium, cook them for 7 minutes, flip, cook them for 7 minutes more, transfer to a plate and keep them warm.
4. Return pan to medium heat, add shallots, stir and cook for 3 minutes.
5. Add stock, stir and cook for 1 minute.
6. Add Worcestershire sauce, mustard, erythritol, cream, rosemary and thyme spring, stir and cook for 8 minutes.
7. Add lemon juice, salt, pepper and the ghee, discard rosemary and thyme, stir well and take off heat.
8. Divide lamb chops on plates, drizzle the sauce over them and serve.
Enjoy!

Nutrition: calories 435, fat 30, fiber 4, carbs 5, protein 32

Tasty Lamb Curry

Preparation time: 10 minutes
Cooking time: 4 hours
Servings: 6

Ingredients:
2 tablespoons ginger, grated
2 garlic cloves, minced
2 teaspoons cardamom
1 red onion, chopped
6 cloves
1 pound lamb meat, cubed
2 teaspoons cumin powder
1 teaspoon garama masala
½ teaspoon chili powder
1 teaspoon turmeric
2 teaspoons coriander, ground
1 pound spinach
14 ounces canned tomatoes, chopped

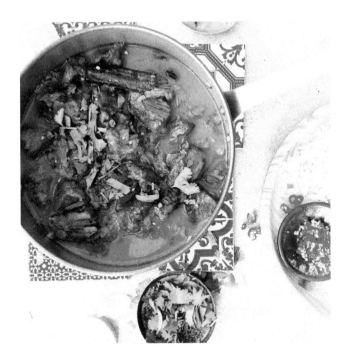

Directions:
1. In your slow cooker, mix lamb with spinach, tomatoes, ginger, garlic, onion, cardamom, cloves, cumin, garam masala, chili, turmeric and coriander, stir, cover and cook on High for 4 hours.
2. Uncover slow cooker, stir your chili, divide into bowls and serve.
Enjoy!

Nutrition: calories 160, fat 6, fiber 3, carbs 7, protein 20

Tasty Lamb Stew

Preparation time: 10 minutes
Cooking time: 3 hours
Servings: 4

Ingredients:
1 yellow onion, chopped
3 carrots, chopped
2 pounds lamb, cubed
1 tomato, chopped
1 garlic clove, minced
2 tablespoons ghee
1 cup beef stock
1 cup white wine
Salt and black pepper to the taste
2 rosemary springs
1 teaspoon thyme, chopped

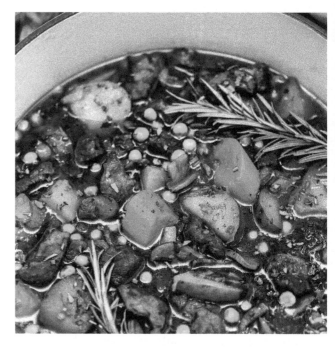

Directions:
1. Heat up a Dutch oven over medium high heat, add oil and heat up.
2. Add lamb, salt and pepper, brown on all sides and transfer to a plate.
3. Add onion to the pot and cook for 2 minutes.
4. Add carrots, tomato, garlic, ghee, stick, wine, salt, pepper, rosemary and thyme, stir and cook for a couple of minutes.
5. Return lamb to pot, stir, reduce heat to medium low, cover and cook for 4 hours.
6. Discard rosemary springs, add more salt and pepper, stir,
divide into bowls and serve.
Enjoy!

Nutrition: calories 700, fat 43, fiber 6, carbs 10, protein 67

Delicious Lamb Casserole

Preparation time: 10 minutes
Cooking time: 1 hour and 40 minutes
Servings: 2

Ingredients:
2 garlic cloves, minced
1 red onion, chopped
1 tablespoon olive oil
1 celery stick, chopped
10 ounces lamb fillet, cut into medium pieces
Salt and black pepper to the taste
1 and ¼ cups lamb stock
2 carrots, chopped
½ tablespoon rosemary, chopped
1 leek, chopped
1 tablespoon mint sauce
1 teaspoon stevia
1 tablespoon tomato puree
½ cauliflower, florets separated
½ celeriac, chopped
2 tablespoons ghee

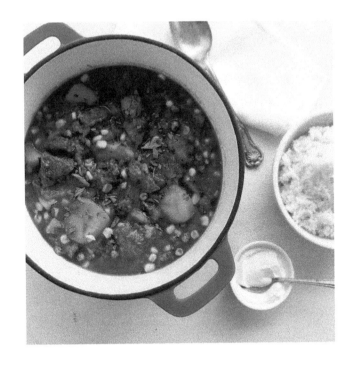

Directions:
1. Heat up a pot with the oil over medium heat, add garlic, onion and celery, stir and cook for 5 minutes.
2. Add lamb pieces, stir and cook for 3 minutes.
3. Add carrot, leek, rosemary, stock, tomato puree, mint sauce and stevia, stir, bring to a boil, cover and cook for 1 hour and 30 minutes.
4. Heat up a pot with water over medium heat, add celeriac, cover and simmer for 10 minutes.
5. Add cauliflower florets, cook for 15 minutes, drain everything and mix with salt, pepper and ghee.
6. Mash using a potato masher and divide mash between plates.
7. Add lamb and veggies mix on top and serve.
Enjoy!

Nutrition: calories 324, fat 4, fiber 5, carbs 8, protein 20

Amazing Lamb

Preparation time: 10 minutes
Cooking time: 8 hours
Servings: 6

Ingredients:
2 pounds lamb leg
Salt and black pepper to the taste
1 tablespoon maple extract
2 tablespoons mustard
¼ cup olive oil
4 thyme spring
6 mint leaves
1 teaspoon garlic, minced
A pinch of rosemary, dried

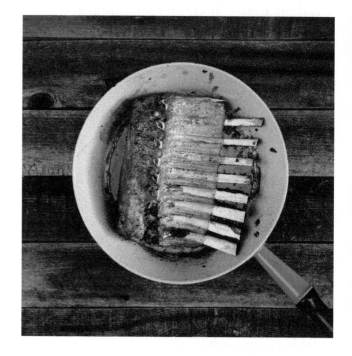

Directions:
1. Put the oil in your slow cooker.
2. Add lamb, salt, pepper, maple extract, mustard, rosemary and garlic, rub well, cover and cook on Low for 7 hours.
3. Add mint and thyme and cook for 1 more hour.
4. Leave lamb to cool down a bit before slicing and serving with pan juices on top. Enjoy!

Nutrition: calories 400, fat 34, fiber 1, carbs 3, protein 26

Lavender Lamb Chops

Preparation time: 10 minutes
Cooking time: 25 minutes
Servings: 4

Ingredients:
2 tablespoons rosemary, chopped
1 and ½ pounds lamb chops
Salt and black pepper to the taste
1 tablespoon lavender, chopped
2 garlic cloves, minced
3 red oranges, cut in halves
2 small pieces of orange peel
A drizzle of olive oil
1 teaspoon ghee

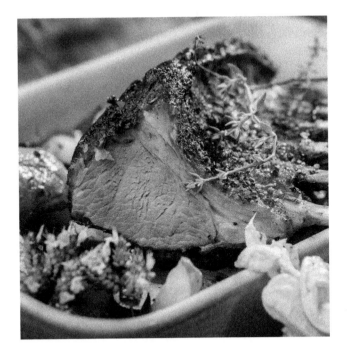

Directions:
1. In a bowl, mix lamb chops with salt, pepper, rosemary, lavender, garlic and orange peel, toss to coat and leave aside for a couple of hours.
2. Grease your kitchen grill with ghee, heat up over medium high heat, place lamb chops on it, cook for 3 minutes, flip, squeeze 1 orange half over them, cook for 3 minutes more, flip them again, cook them for 2 minutes and squeeze another orange half over them.
3. Place lamb chops on a plate and keep them warm for now..
4. Add remaining orange halves on preheated grill, cook them for
3 minutes, flip and cook them for another 3 minutes.
5. Divide lamb chops between plates, add orange halves on the side, drizzle some olive oil over them and serve.
Enjoy!

Nutrition: calories 250, fat 5, fiber 1, carbs 5, protein 8

Crusted Lamb Chops

Preparation time: 10 minutes
Cooking time: 15 minutes
Servings: 4

Ingredients:
2 lamb racks, cut into chops
Salt and black pepper to the taste
3 tablespoons paprika
¾ cup cumin powder
1 teaspoon chili powder

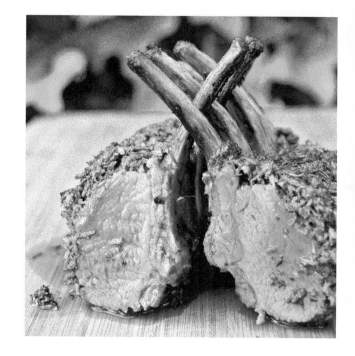

Directions:
1. In a bowl, mix paprika with cumin, chili, salt and pepper and stir.
2. Add lamb chops and rub them well.
3. Heat up your grill over medium temperature, add lamb chops, cook for 5 minutes, flip and cook for 5 minutes more.
4. Flip them again, cook for 2 minutes and then for 2 minutes more on the other side again. Enjoy!

Nutrition: calories 200, fat 5, fiber 2, carbs 4, protein 8

Lamb And Orange Dressing

Preparation time: 10 minutes
Cooking time: 4 hours
Servings: 4

Ingredients:
2 lamb shanks
Salt and black pepper to the taste
1 garlic head, peeled
4 tablespoons olive oil
Juice of ½ lemon
Zest from ½ lemon
½ teaspoon oregano, dried

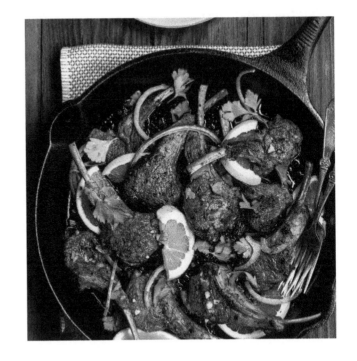

Directions:
1. In your slow cooker, mix lamb with salt and pepper.
2. Add garlic, cover and cook on High for 4 hours.
3. Meanwhile, in a bowl, mix lemon juice with lemon zest, some salt and pepper, the olive oil and oregano and whisk very well.
4. Uncover your slow cooker, shred lamb meat and discard bone and divide between plates.
5. Drizzle the lemon dressing all over and serve.
Enjoy!

Nutrition: calories 160, fat 7, fiber 3, carbs 5, protein 12

Lamb Riblets And Tasty Mint Pesto

Preparation time: 1 hour
Cooking time: 2 hours
Servings: 4

Ingredients:
1 cup parsley
1 cup mint
1 small yellow onion, roughly chopped
1/3 cup pistachios
1 teaspoon lemon zest
5 tablespoons avocado oil
Salt to the taste
2 pounds lamb riblets
½ onion, chopped
5 garlic cloves, minced
Juice from 1 orange

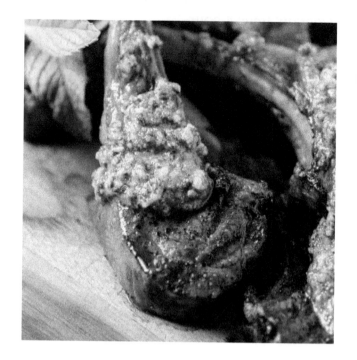

Directions:
1. In your food processor, mix parsley with mint, 1 small onion, pistachios, lemon zest, salt and avocado oil and blend very well.
2. Rub lamb with this mix, place in a bowl, cover and leave in the fridge for 1 hour.
3. Transfer lamb to a baking dish, add garlic and ½ onion to the dish as well, drizzle orange juice and bake in the oven at 250 degrees F for 2 hours.
4. Divide between plates and serve.
Enjoy!

Nutrition: calories 200, fat 4, fiber 1, carbs 5, protein 7

Lamb With Fennel And Figs

Preparation time: 10 minutes
Cooking time: 40 minutes
Servings: 4

Ingredients:
12 ounces lamb racks
2 fennel bulbs, sliced
Salt and black pepper to the taste
2 tablespoons olive oil
4 figs, cut in halves
1/8 cup apple cider vinegar
1 tablespoon swerve

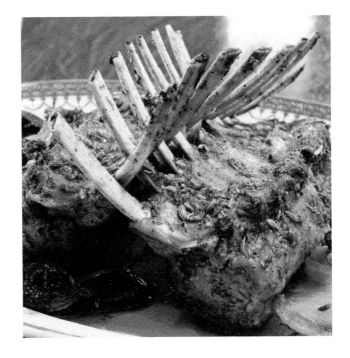

Directions:
1. In a bowl, mix fennel with figs, vinegar, swerve and oil, toss to coat well and transfer to a baking dish.
2. Season with salt and pepper, introduce in the oven at 400 degrees F and bake for 15 minutes.
3. Season lamb with salt and pepper, place into a heated pan over medium high heat and cook for a couple of minutes.
4. Add lamb to the baking dish with the fennel and figs, introduce in the oven and bake for 20 minutes more.
5. Divide everything between plates and serve.
Enjoy!

Nutrition: calories 230, fat 3, fiber 3, carbs 5, protein 10

Baked Veal And Cabbage

Preparation time: 10 minutes
Cooking time: 40 minutes
Servings: 4

Ingredients:
17 ounces veal, cut into cubes
1 cabbage, shredded
Salt and black pepper to the taste
3.4 ounces ham, roughly chopped
1 small yellow onion, chopped
2 garlic cloves, minced
1 tablespoon ghee
½ cup parmesan, grated
½ cup sour cream

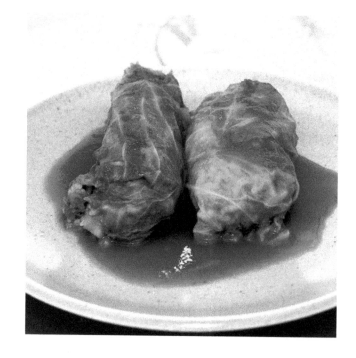

Directions:
1. Heat up a pot with the ghee over medium high heat, add onion, stir and cook for 2 minutes.
2. Add garlic, stir and cook for 1 minute more.
3. Add ham and veal, stir and cook until they brown a bit.
4. Add cabbage, stir and cook until it softens and the meat is tender.
5. Add cream, salt, pepper and cheese, stir gently, introduce in the oven at 350 degrees F and bake for 20 minutes.
6. Divide between plates and serve.
Enjoy!

Nutrition: calories 230, fat 7, fiber 4, carbs 6, protein 29

Delicious Beef Bourguignon

Preparation time: 3 hours and 10 minutes
Cooking time: 5 hours and 15 minutes
Servings: 8

Ingredients:
3 tablespoons olive oil
2 tablespoons onion, chopped
1 tablespoon parsley flakes
1 and ½ cups red wine
1 teaspoon thyme, dried
Salt and black pepper to the taste
1 bay leaf
1/3 cup almond flour
4 pounds beef, cubed
24 small white onions
8 bacon slices, chopped, 2 garlic cloves, minced
1 pound mushrooms, roughly chopped

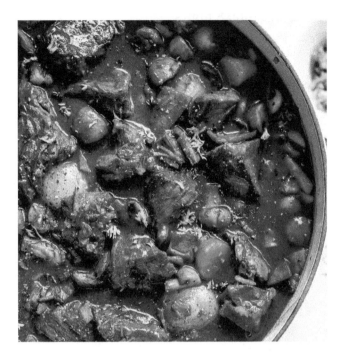

Directions:
1. In a bowl, mix wine with olive oil, minced onion, thyme, parsley, salt, pepper and bay leaf and whisk well.
2. Add beef cubes, stir and leave aside for 3 hours.
3. Drain meat and reserve 1 cup of marinade.
4. Add flour over meat and toss to coat.
5. Heat up a pan over medium high heat, add bacon, stir and cook until it browns a bit.
6. Add onions, stir and cook for 3 minutes more.
7. Add garlic, stir, cook for 1 minute and transfer everything to a slow cooker.
8. Also add meat to the slow cooker and stir.
9. Heat up the pan with the bacon fat over medium high heat, add mushrooms and white onions, stir and sauté them for a couple
of minutes.
10. Add these to the slow cooker as well, also add reserved marinade, some salt and pepper, cover and cook on High for 5
hours.
11. Divide between plates and serve.
Enjoy!

Nutrition: calories 435, fat 16, fiber 1, carbs 7, protein 45

Roasted Beef

Preparation time: 10 minutes
Cooking time: 8 hours
Servings: 8

Ingredients:
5 pounds beef roast
Salt and black pepper to the taste
½ teaspoon celery salt
2 teaspoons chili powder
1 tablespoon avocado oil
1 tablespoon sweet paprika
A pinch of cayenne pepper
½ teaspoon garlic powder
½ cup beef stock
1 tablespoon garlic, minced
¼ teaspoon dry mustard

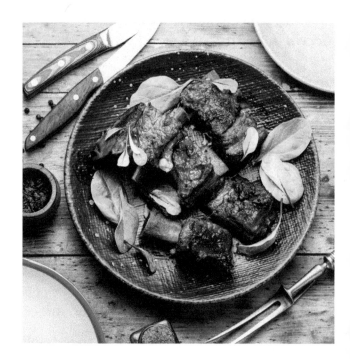

Directions:
1. Heat up a pan with the oil over medium high heat, add beef roast and brown it on all sides.
2. In a bowl, mix paprika with chili powder, celery salt, salt, pepper, cayenne, garlic powder and mustard powder and stir.
3. Add roast, rub well and transfer it to a Crockpot.
4. Add beef stock and garlic over roast and cook on Low for 8 hours.
5. Transfer beef to a cutting board, leave it to cool down a bit, slice and divide between plates.
6. Strain juices from the pot, drizzle over meat and serve.
Enjoy!

Nutrition: calories 180, fat 5, fiber 1, carbs 5, protein 25

Amazing Beef Stew

Preparation time: 10 minutes
Cooking time: 4 hours and 10 minutes
Servings: 4

Ingredients:
8 ounces pancetta, chopped
4 pounds beef, cubed
4 garlic cloves, minced
2 brown onions, chopped
2 tablespoons olive oil
4 tablespoons red vinegar
4 cups beef stock
2 tablespoons tomato paste
2 cinnamon sticks
3 lemon peel strips
A handful parsley, chopped
4 thyme springs
2 tablespoons ghee
Salt and black pepper to the taste

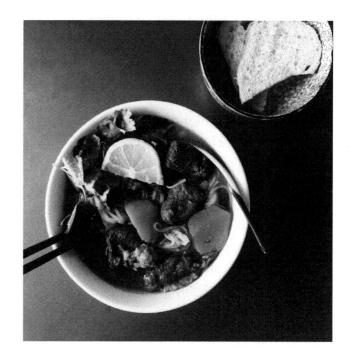

Directions:
1. Heat up a pan with the oil over medium high heat, add pancetta, onion and garlic, stir and cook for 5 minutes. Add beef, stir and cook until it browns.
2. Add vinegar, salt, pepper, stock, tomato paste, cinnamon, lemon peel, thyme and ghee, stir, cook for 3 minutes and transfer everything to your slow cooker.
3. Cover and cook on High for 4 hours.
4. Discard cinnamon, lemon peel and thyme, add parsley, stir and divide into bowls.
5. Serve hot.
Enjoy!

Nutrition: calories 250, fat 6, fiber 1, carbs 7, protein 33

Delicious Pork Stew

Preparation time: 10 minutes
Cooking time: 1 hour and 20 minutes
Servings: 12

Ingredients:
2 tablespoons coconut oil
4 pounds pork, cubed
Salt and black pepper to the taste
2 tablespoons ghee
3 garlic cloves, minced
¾ cup beef stock
¾ cup apple cider vinegar
3 carrots, chopped
1 cabbage head, shredded
½ cup green onion, chopped
1 cup whipping cream

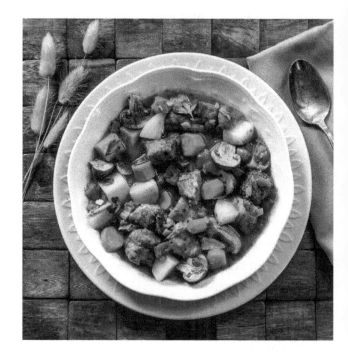

Directions:
1. Heat up a pan with the ghee and the oil over medium high heat, add pork and brown it for a few minutes on each side.
2. Add vinegar and stock, stir well and bring to a simmer.
3. Add cabbage, garlic, salt and pepper, stir, cover and cook for 1 hour.
4. Add carrots and green onions, stir and cook for 15 minutes more.
5. Add whipping cream, stir for 1 minute, divide between plates and serve.
Enjoy!

Nutrition: calories 400, fat 25, fiber 3, carbs 6, protein 43

Delicious Sausage Stew

Preparation time: 10 minutes
Cooking time: 20 minutes
Servings: 9

Ingredients:
1 pound smoked sausage, sliced
1 green bell pepper, chopped
2 yellow onions, chopped
Salt and black pepper to the taste
1 cup parsley, chopped
8 green onions, chopped
¼ cup avocado oil
1 cup beef stock
6 garlic cloves
28 ounces canned tomatoes, chopped
16 ounces okra, chopped
8 ounces tomato sauce
2 tablespoons coconut aminos
1 tablespoon gluten free hot sauce

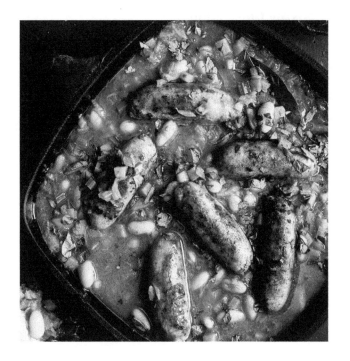

Directions:
1. Heat up a pot with the oil over medium high heat, add sausages, stir and cook for 2 minutes.
2. Add onion, bell pepper, green onions, parsley, salt and pepper, stir and cook for 2 minutes more.
3. Add stock, garlic, tomatoes, okra, tomato sauce, coconut aminos and hot sauce, stir, bring to a simmer and cook for 15 minutes.
4. Add more salt and pepper, stir, divide into bowls and serve.
Enjoy!

Nutrition: calories 274, fat 20, fiber 4, carbs 7, protein 10

Burgundy Beef Stew

Preparation time: 10 minutes
Cooking time: 3 hours
Servings: 7

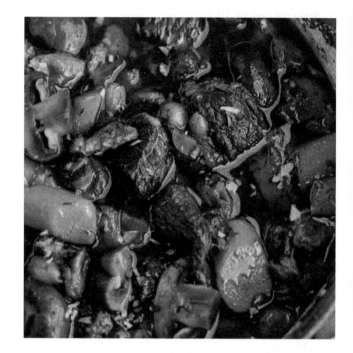

Ingredients:
2 pounds beef chuck roast, cubed
15 ounces canned tomatoes, chopped
4 carrots, chopped
Salt and black pepper to the taste
½ pounds mushrooms, sliced
2 celery ribs, chopped
2 yellow onions, chopped
1 cup beef stock
1 tablespoon thyme, chopped
½ teaspoon mustard powder
3 tablespoons almond flour
1 cup water

Directions:
1. Heat up an oven proof pot over medium high heat, add beef cubes, stir and brown them for a couple of minutes on each side.
2. Add tomatoes, mushrooms, onions, carrots, celery, salt, pepper mustard, stock and thyme and stir.
3. In a bowl mix water with flour and stir well. Add this to the pot, stir well, introduce in the oven and bake at 325 degrees F for 3 hours.
4. Stir every half an hour.
5. Divide into bowls and serve.
Enjoy!

Nutrition: calories 275, fat 13, fiber 4, carbs 7, protein 28

Cuban Beef Stew

Preparation time: 10 minutes
Cooking time: 6 hours
Servings: 8

Ingredients:
2 yellow onions, chopped
2 tablespoons avocado oil
2 pounds beef roast, cubed
2 green bell peppers, chopped
1 habanero pepper, chopped
4 jalapenos, chopped
14 ounces canned tomatoes, chopped
2 tablespoons cilantro, chopped
6 garlic cloves, minced
½ cup water
Salt and black pepper to the taste
1 and ½ teaspoons cumin, ground
4 teaspoons bouillon granules
½ cup black olives, pitted and chopped
1 teaspoon oregano, dried

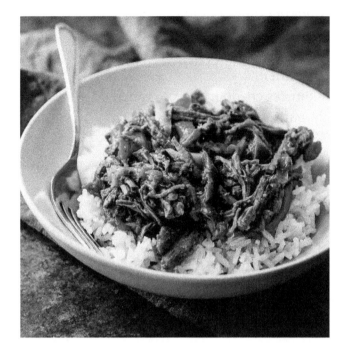

Directions:
1. Heat up a pan with the oil over medium high heat, add beef, brown it on all sides and transfer to a slow cooker.
2. Add green bell peppers, onions, jalapenos, habanero pepper, tomatoes, garlic, water, bouillon, cilantro, oregano, cumin, salt and pepper and stir.
3. Cover slow cooker and cook on Low for 6 hours.
4. Add olives, stir, divide into bowls and serve.
Enjoy!

Nutrition: calories 305, fat 14, fiber 4, carbs 8, protein 25

Ham Stew

Preparation time: 10 minutes
Cooking time: 4 hours
Servings: 6

Ingredients:
8 ounces cheddar cheese, grated
14 ounces chicken stock
½ teaspoon garlic powder
½ teaspoon onion powder
Salt and black pepper to the taste
4 garlic cloves, minced
¼ cup heavy cream
3 cups ham, chopped
16 ounces cauliflower florets

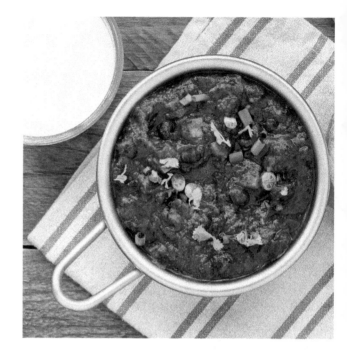

Directions:
1. In your Crockpot, mix ham with stock, cheese, cauliflower, garlic powder, onion powder, salt, pepper, garlic and heavy cream, stir, cover and cook on High for 4 hours.
2. Stir, divide into bowls and serve.
Enjoy!

Nutrition: calories 320, fat 20, fiber 3, carbs 6, protein 23

VEGETABLE

Amazing Broccoli And Cauliflower Cream

Preparation time: 10 minutes
Cooking time: 15 minutes
Servings: 5

Ingredients:
1 cauliflower head, florets separated
1 broccoli head, florets separated
Salt and black pepper to the taste
2 garlic cloves, minced
2 bacon slices, chopped
2 tablespoons ghee

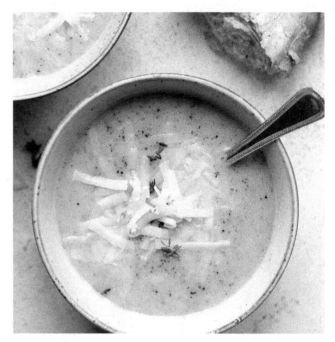

Directions:
1. Heat up a pot with the ghee over medium high heat, add garlic and bacon, stir and cook for 3 minutes.
2. Add cauliflower and broccoli florets, stir and cook for 2
minutes more.
3. Add water to cover them, cover pot and simmer for 10 minutes.
4. Add salt and pepper, stir again and blend soup using an immersion blender.
5. Simmer for a couple more minutes over medium heat, ladle into bowls and serve.
Enjoy!

Nutrition: calories 230, fat 3, fiber 3, carbs 6, protein 10

Broccoli Stew

Preparation time: 10 minutes
Cooking time: 40 minutes
Servings: 4

Ingredients:
1 broccoli head, florets separated
2 teaspoons coriander seeds
A drizzle of olive oil
1 yellow onion, chopped
Salt and black pepper to the taste
A pinch of red pepper, crushed
1 small ginger piece, chopped
1 garlic clove, minced
28 ounces canned tomatoes, pureed

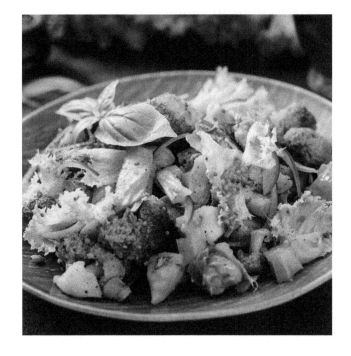

Directions:
1. Put water in a pot, add salt, bring to a boil over medium high heat, add broccoli florets, steam them for 2 minutes, transfer them to a bowl filled with ice water, drain them and leave aside.
2. Heat up a pan over medium high heat, add coriander seeds, toast them for 4 minutes, transfer to a grinder, ground them and leave aside as well.
3. Heat up a pot with the oil over medium heat, add onions, salt, pepper and red pepper, stir and cook for 7 minutes.
4. Add ginger, garlic and coriander seeds, stir and cook for 3 minutes.
5. Add tomatoes, bring to a boil and simmer for 10 minutes.
6. Add broccoli, stir and cook your stew for 12 minutes.
7. Divide into bowls and serve.
Enjoy!

Nutrition: calories 150, fat 4, fiber 2, carbs 5, protein 12

Amazing Watercress Soup

Preparation time: 10 minutes
Cooking time: 10 minutes
Servings: 4

Ingredients:
6 cup chicken stock
¼ cup sherry
2 teaspoons coconut aminos
6 and ½ cups watercress
Salt and black pepper to the taste
2 teaspoons sesame seed
3 shallots, chopped
3 egg whites, whisked

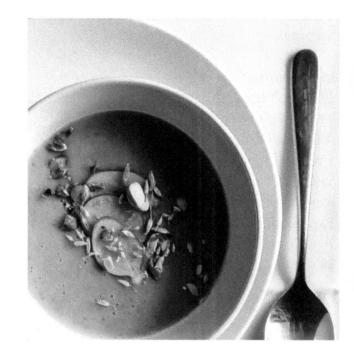

Directions:
1. Put stock into a pot, mix with salt, pepper, sherry and coconut aminos, stir and bring to a boil over medium high heat.
2. Add shallots, watercress and egg whites, stir, bring to a boil, divide into bowls and serve with sesame seeds sprinkled on top.
Enjoy!

Nutrition: calories 50, fat 1, fiber 0, carbs 1, protein 5

Delicious Bok Choy Soup

Preparation time: 10 minutes
Cooking time: 15 minutes
Servings: 4

Ingredients:
3 cups beef stock
1 yellow onion, chopped
1 bunch bok choy, chopped
1 and ½ cups mushrooms, chopped
Salt and black pepper to the taste
½ tablespoon red pepper flakes
3 tablespoons coconut aminos
3 tablespoons parmesan, grated
2 tablespoons Worcestershire sauce
2 bacon strips, chopped

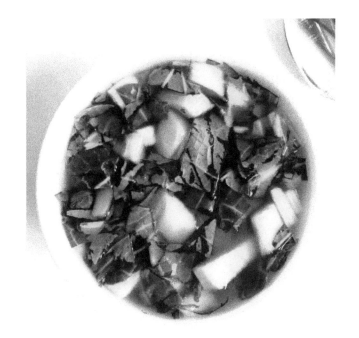

Directions:
1. Heat up a pot over medium high heat, add bacon, stir, cook until it until it's crispy, transfer to paper towels and drain grease.
2. Heat up the pot again over medium heat, add mushrooms and onions, stir and cook for 5 minutes.
3. Add stock, bok choy, coconut aminos, salt, pepper, pepper flakes and Worcestershire sauce, stir, cover and cook until bok choy is tender.
4. Ladle soup into bowls, sprinkle parmesan and bacon and serve.
Enjoy!

Nutrition: calories 100, fat 3, fiber 1, carbs 2, protein 6

Bok Choy Stir Fry

Preparation time: 10 minutes
Cooking time: 7 minutes
Servings: 2

Ingredients:
2 garlic cloves, minced
2 cup bok choy, chopped
2 bacon slices, chopped
Salt and black pepper to the taste
A drizzle of avocado oil

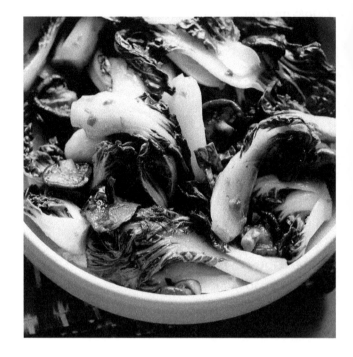

Directions:
1. Heat up a pan with the oil over medium heat, add bacon, stir and brown until it's crispy, transfer to paper towels and drain grease.
2. Return pan to medium heat, add garlic and bok choy, stir and cook for 4 minutes.
3. Add salt, pepper and return bacon, stir, cook for 1 minute more, divide between plates and serve.
Enjoy!

Nutrition: calories 50, fat 1, fiber 1, carbs 2, protein 2

Cream Of Celery

Preparation time: 10 minutes
Cooking time: 40 minutes
Servings: 4

Ingredients:
1 bunch celery, chopped
Salt and black pepper to the taste
3 bay leaves
½ garlic head, chopped
2 yellow onions, chopped
4 cups chicken stock
¾ cup heavy cream
2 tablespoons ghee

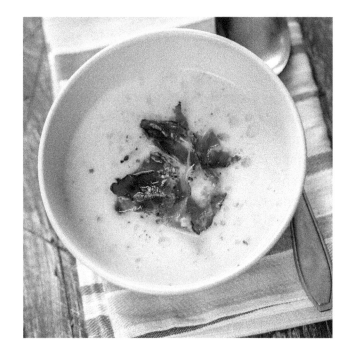

Directions:
1. Heat up a pot with the ghee over medium high heat, add onions, salt and pepper, stir and cook for 5 minutes.
2. Add bay leaves, garlic and celery, stir and cook for 15 minutes.
3. Add stock, more salt and pepper, stir, cover pot, reduce heat and simmer for 20 minutes.
4. Add cream, stir and blend everything using an immersion blender.
5. Ladle into soup bowls and serve.
Enjoy!

Nutrition: calories 150, fat 3, fiber 1, carbs 2, protein 6

Delightful Celery Soup

Preparation time: 10 minutes
Cooking time: 25 minutes
Servings: 8

Ingredients:
26 ounces celery leaves and stalks, chopped
1 tablespoon onion flakes
Salt and black pepper to the taste
3 teaspoons fenugreek powder
3 teaspoons veggie stock powder
10 ounces sour cream

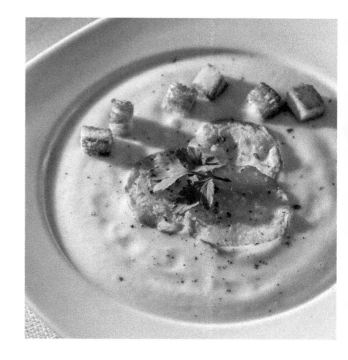

Directions:
1. Put celery into a pot, add water to cover, add onion flakes, salt, pepper, stock powder and fenugreek powder, stir, bring to a boil over medium heat and simmer for 20 minutes.
2. Use an immersion blender to make your cream, add sour cream, more salt and pepper and blend again.
3. Heat up soup again over medium heat, ladle into bowls and serve.
Enjoy!

Nutrition: calories 140, fat 2, fiber 1, carbs 5, protein 10

Amazing Celery Stew

Preparation time: 10 minutes
Cooking time: 30 minutes
Servings: 6

Ingredients:
1 celery bunch, roughly chopped
1 yellow onion, chopped
1 bunch green onion, chopped
4 garlic cloves, minced
Salt and black pepper to the taste
1 parsley bunch, chopped
2 mint bunches, chopped
3 dried Persian lemons, pricked with a fork
2 cups water
2 teaspoons chicken bouillon
4 tablespoons olive oil

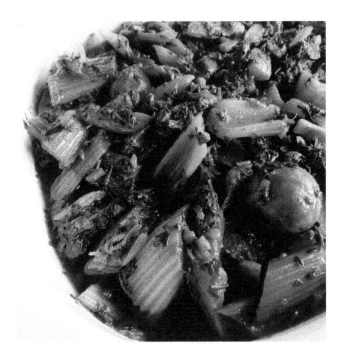

Directions:
1. Heat up a pot with the oil over medium high heat, add onion, green onions and garlic, stir and cook for 6 minutes.
2. Add celery, Persian lemons, chicken bouillon, salt, pepper and water, stir, cover pot and simmer on medium heat for 20 minutes.
3. Add parsley and mint, stir and cook for 10 minutes more.
4. Divide into bowls and serve.
Enjoy!

Nutrition: calories 170, fat 7, fiber 4, carbs 6, protein 10

Spinach Soup

Preparation time: 10 minutes
Cooking time: 15 minutes
Servings: 8

Ingredients:
2 tablespoons ghee
20 ounces spinach, chopped
1 teaspoon garlic, minced
Salt and black pepper to the taste
45 ounces chicken stock
½ teaspoon nutmeg, ground
2 cups heavy cream
1 yellow onion, chopped

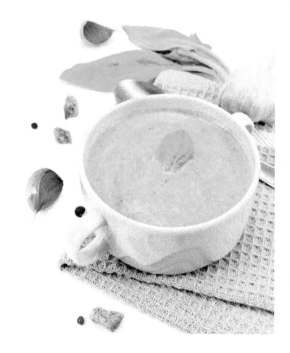

Directions:
1. Heat up a pot with the ghee over medium heat, add onion, stir and cook for 4 minutes.
2. Add garlic, stir and cook for 1 minute.
3. Add spinach and stock, stir and cook for 5 minutes.
4. Blend soup with an immersion blender and heat up the soup again.
5. Add salt, pepper, nutmeg and cream, stir and cook for 5 minutes more.
6. Ladle into bowls and serve.
Enjoy!

Nutrition: calories 245, fat 24, fiber 3, carbs 4, protein 6

Delicious Mustard Greens Sauté

Preparation time: 10 minutes
Cooking time: 20 minutes
Servings: 4

Ingredients:
2 garlic cloves, minced
1 tablespoon olive oil
2 and ½ pounds collard greens, chopped
1 teaspoon lemon juice
1 tablespoon ghee
Salt and black pepper to the taste

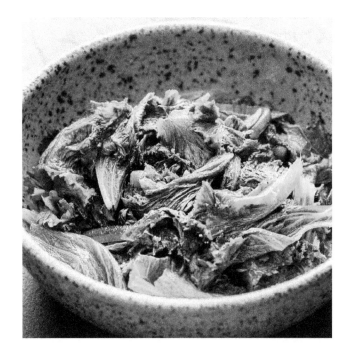

Directions:
1. Put some water in a pot, add salt and bring to a simmer over medium heat.
2. Add greens, cover and cook for 15 minutes.
3. Drain collard greens well, press out liquid and put them into a bowl.
4. Heat up a pan with the oil and the ghee over medium high heat, add collard greens, salt, pepper and garlic.
5. Stir well and cook for 5 minutes.
6. Add more salt and pepper if needed, drizzle lemon juice, stir, divide between plates and serve. Enjoy!

Nutrition: calories 151, fat 6, fiber 3, carbs 7, protein 8

Tasty Collards Greens And Ham

Preparation time: 10 minutes
Cooking time: 1 hour and 40 minutes
Servings: 4

Ingredients:
4 ounces ham, boneless, cooked and chopped
1 tablespoon olive oil
2 pounds collard greens, cut in medium strips
1 teaspoon red pepper flakes, crushed
Salt and black pepper to the taste
2 cups chicken stock
1 yellow onion, chopped
4 ounces dry white wine
1 ounce salt pork
¼ cup apple cider vinegar
½ cup ghee, melted

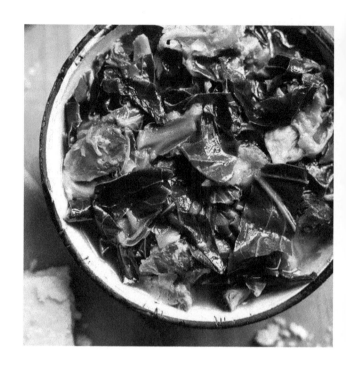

Directions:
1. Heat up a pan with the oil over medium high heat, add ham and onion, stir and cook for 4 minutes.
2. Add salt pork, collard greens, stock, vinegar and wine, stir and bring to a boil.
3. Reduce heat, cover pan and cook for 1 hour and 30 minutes stirring from time to time.
4. Add ghee, discard salt pork, stir, cook everything for 10 minutes, divide between plates and serve.
Enjoy!

Nutrition: calories 150, fat 12, fiber 2, carbs 4, protein 8

Tasty Collard Greens And Tomatoes

Preparation time: 10 minutes
Cooking time: 12 minutes
Servings: 5

Ingredients:
1 pound collard greens
3 bacon strips, chopped
¼ cup cherry tomatoes, halved
1 tablespoon apple cider vinegar
2 tablespoons chicken stock
Salt and black pepper to the taste

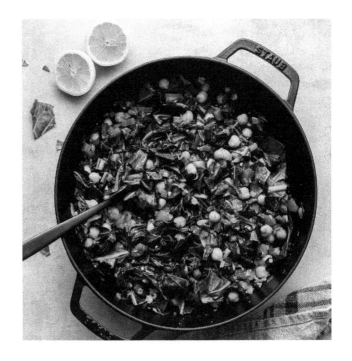

Directions:
1. Heat up a pan over medium heat, add bacon, stir and cook until it browns.
2. Add tomatoes, collard greens, vinegar, stock, salt and pepper, stir and cook for 8 minutes.
3. Add more salt and pepper, stir again gently, divide between plates and serve.
Enjoy!

Nutrition: calories 120, fat 8, fiber 1, carbs 3, protein 7

Simple Mustard Greens Dish

Preparation time: 5 minutes
Cooking time: 15 minutes
Servings: 4

Ingredients:
2 garlic cloves, minced
1 pound mustard greens, torn
1 tablespoon olive oil
½ cup yellow onion, sliced
Salt and black pepper to the taste
3 tablespoons veggie stock
¼ teaspoon dark sesame oil

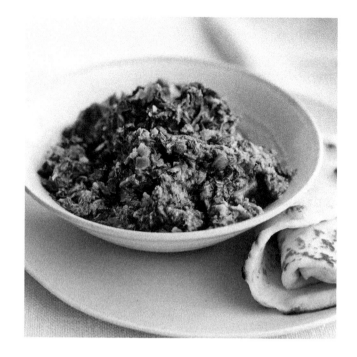

Directions:
1. Heat up a pan with the oil over medium heat, add onions, stir and brown them for 10 minutes.
2. Add garlic, stir and cook for 1 minute.
3. Add stock, greens, salt and pepper, stir and cook for 5 minutes more.
4. Add more salt and pepper and the sesame oil, toss to coat, divide between plates and serve. Enjoy!

Nutrition: calories 120, fat 3, fiber 1, carbs 3, protein 6

Delicious Collard Greens And Poached Eggs

Preparation time: 10 minutes
Cooking time: 15 minutes
Servings: 6

Ingredients:
1 tablespoon chipotle in adobo, mashed
6 eggs
3 tablespoons ghee
1 yellow onion, chopped
2 garlic cloves, minced
6 bacon slices, chopped
3 bunches collard greens, chopped
½ cup chicken stock
Salt and black pepper to the taste
1 tablespoon lime juice
Some grated cheddar cheese

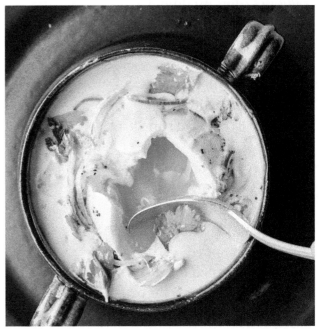

Directions:
1. Heat up a pan over medium high heat, add bacon, cook until it's crispy, transfer to paper towels, drain grease and leave aside.
2. Heat up the pan again over medium heat, add garlic and onion, stir and cook for 2 minutes.
3. Return bacon to the pan, stir and cook for 3 minutes more.
4. Add chipotle in adobo paste, collard greens, salt and pepper, stir and cook for 10 minutes.
5. Add stock and lime juice and stir.
6. Make 6 holes in collard greens mix, divide ghee in them, crack an egg in each hole, cover pan and cook until eggs are done.
7. Divide this between plates and serve with cheddar cheese sprinkled on top.
Enjoy!

Nutrition: calories 245, fat 20, fiber 1, carbs 5, protein 12

Collard Greens Soup

Preparation time: 10 minutes
Cooking time: 40 minutes
Servings: 12

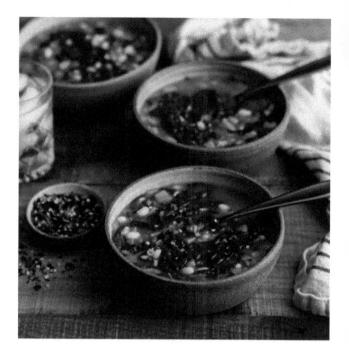

Ingredients:
1 teaspoon chili powder
1 tablespoon avocado oil
2 teaspoons smoked paprika
1 teaspoon cumin
1 yellow onion, chopped
A pinch of red pepper flakes
10 cups water
3 celery stalks, chopped
3 carrots, chopped
15 ounces canned tomatoes, chopped
2 tablespoons tamari sauce
6 ounces canned tomato paste
2 tablespoons lemon juice
Salt and black pepper to the taste
6 cups collard greens, stems discarded
1 tablespoon swerve
1 teaspoon garlic granules
1 tablespoon herb seasoning

Directions:
1. Heat up a pot with the oil over medium high heat, add cumin, pepper flakes, paprika and chili powder and stir well.
2. Add celery, onion and carrots, stir and cook for 10 minutes.
3. Add tamari sauce, tomatoes, tomato paste, water, lemon juice, salt, pepper, herb seasoning, swerve, garlic granules and collard greens, stir, bring to a boil, cover and cook for 30 minutes.
4. Stir again, ladle into bowls and serve.
Enjoy!

Nutrition: calories 150, fat 3, fiber 2, carbs 4, protein 8

Spring Green Soup

Preparation time: 10 minutes
Cooking time: 30 minutes
Servings: 4

Ingredients:
2 cups mustard greens, chopped
2 cups collard greens, chopped
3 quarts veggie stock
1 yellow onion, chopped
Salt and black pepper to the taste
2 tablespoons coconut aminos
2 teaspoons ginger, grated

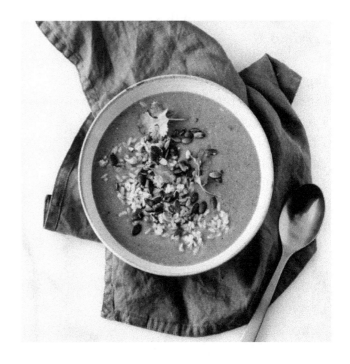

Directions:
1. Put the stock into a pot and bring to a simmer over medium high heat.
2. Add mustard and collard greens, onion, salt, pepper, coconut aminos and ginger, stir, cover pot and cook for 30 minutes.
3. Blend soup using an immersion blender, add more salt and pepper, heat up over medium heat, ladle into soup bowls and serve.
Enjoy!

Nutrition: calories 140, fat 2, fiber 1, carbs 3, protein 7

Mustard Greens And Spinach Soup

Preparation time: 10 minutes
Cooking time: 15 minutes
Servings: 6

Ingredients:
½ teaspoon fenugreek seeds
1 teaspoon cumin seeds
1 tablespoon avocado oil
1 teaspoon coriander seeds
1 cup yellow onion, chopped
1 tablespoon garlic, minced
1 tablespoon ginger, grated
½ teaspoon turmeric, ground
5 cups mustard greens, chopped
3 cups coconut milk
1 tablespoon jalapeno, chopped
5 cups spinach, torn
Salt and black pepper to the taste
2 teaspoons ghee
½ teaspoon paprika

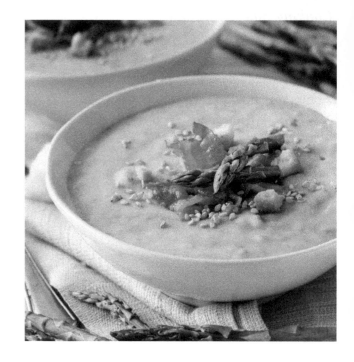

Directions:
1. Heat up a pot with the oil over medium high heat, add coriander, fenugreek and cumin seeds, stir and brown them for 2 minutes.
2. Add onions, stir and cook for 3 minutes more.
3. Add half of the garlic, jalapenos, ginger and turmeric, stir and cook for 3 minutes more.
4. Add mustard greens and spinach, stir and sauté everything for 10 minutes.
5. Add milk, salt and pepper and blend soup using an immersion blender.
6. Heat up a pan with the ghee over medium heat, add garlic and paprika, stir well and take off heat.
7. Heat up the soup over medium heat, ladle into soup bowls, drizzle ghee and paprika all over and soup.
Enjoy!

Nutrition: calories 143, fat 6, fiber 3, carbs 7, protein 7

Roasted Asparagus

Preparation time: 10 minutes
Cooking time: 10 minutes
Servings: 3

Ingredients:
1 asparagus bunch, trimmed
3 teaspoons avocado oil
A splash of lemon juice
Salt and black pepper to the taste
1 tablespoon oregano, chopped

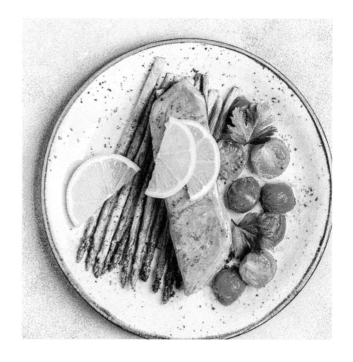

Directions:
1. Spread asparagus spears on a lined baking sheet, season with salt and pepper, drizzle oil and lemon juice, sprinkle oregano and toss to coat well.
2. Introduce in the oven at 425 degrees F and bake for 10 minutes. Divide between plates and serve.
Enjoy!

Nutrition: calories 130, fat 1, fiber 1, carbs 2, protein 3

Simple Asparagus Fries

Preparation time: 10 minutes
Cooking time: 10 minutes
Servings: 2

Ingredients:
¼ cup parmesan, grated
16 asparagus spears, trimmed
1 egg, whisked
½ teaspoon onion powder
2 ounces pork rinds

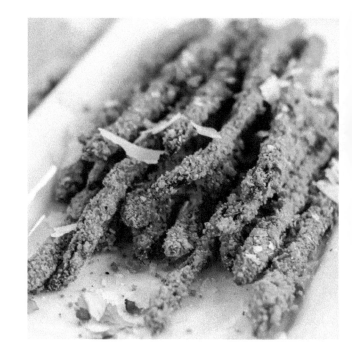

Directions:
1. Crush pork rinds and put them in a bowl.
2. Add onion powder and cheese and stir everything.
3. Roll asparagus spears in egg, then dip them in pork rind mix and arrange them all on a lined baking sheet.
4. Introduce in the oven at 425 degrees F and bake for 10 minutes.
5. Divide between plates and serve them with some sour cream on the side.
Enjoy!

Nutrition: calories 120, fat 2, fiber 2, carbs 5, protein 8

Amazing Asparagus And Browned Butter

Preparation time: 10 minutes
Cooking time: 15 minutes
Servings: 4

Ingredients:
5 ounces butter
1 tablespoon avocado oil
1 and ½ pounds asparagus, trimmed
1 and ½ tablespoons lemon juice
A pinch of cayenne pepper
8 tablespoons sour cream
Salt and black pepper to the taste
3 ounces parmesan, grated
4 eggs

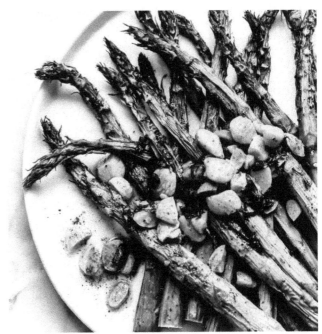

Directions:
1. Heat up a pan with 2 ounces butter over medium high heat, add eggs, some salt and pepper, stir and scramble them.
2. Transfer eggs to a blender, add parmesan, sour cream, salt, pepper and cayenne pepper and blend everything well.
3. Heat up a pan with the oil over medium high heat, add asparagus, salt and pepper, roast for a few minutes, transfer to a plate and leave them aside.
4. Heat up the pan again with the rest of the butter over medium high heat, stir until it's brown, take off heat, add lemon juice and stir well.
5. Heat up the butter again, return asparagus, toss to coat, heat up well and divide between plates.
6. Add blended eggs on top and serve.
Enjoy!

Nutrition: calories 160, fat 7, fiber 2, carbs 6, protein 10

Asparagus Frittata

Preparation time: 10 minutes
Cooking time: 15 minutes
Servings: 4

Ingredients:
¼ cup yellow onion, chopped
A drizzle of olive oil
1 pound asparagus spears, cut into 1 inch pieces
Salt and black pepper to the taste
4 eggs, whisked
1 cup cheddar cheese, grated

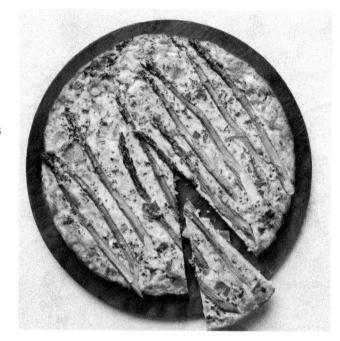

Directions:
1. Heat up a pan with the oil over medium high heat, add onions, stir and cook for 3 minutes.
2. Add asparagus, stir and cook for 6 minutes.
3. Add eggs, stir a bit and cook for 3 minutes.
4. Add salt, pepper and sprinkle the cheese, introduce in the oven and broil for 3 minutes.
5. Divide frittata between plates and serve.
Enjoy!

Nutrition: calories 200, fat 12, fiber 2, carbs 5, protein 14

Creamy Asparagus

Preparation time: 10 minutes
Cooking time: 15 minutes
Servings: 3

Ingredients:
10 ounces asparagus spears, cut into medium pieces and steamed
Salt and black pepper to the taste
2 tablespoons parmesan, grated
1/3 cup Monterey jack cheese, shredded
2 tablespoons mustard
2 ounces cream cheese
1/3 cup heavy cream
3 tablespoons bacon, cooked and crumbled

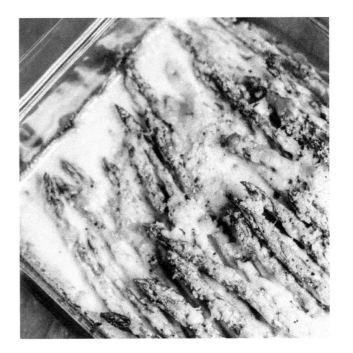

Directions:
1. Heat up a pan with the mustard, heavy cream and cream cheese over medium heat and stir well.
2. Add Monterey Jack cheese and parmesan, stir and cook until it melts.
3. Add half of the bacon and the asparagus, stir and cook for 3 minutes.
4. Add the rest of the bacon, salt and pepper, stir, cook for 5 minutes, divide between plates and serve.
Enjoy!

Nutrition: calories 256, fat 23, fiber 2, carbs 5, protein 13

Delicious Sprouts Salad

Preparation time: 10 minutes
Cooking time: 0 minutes
Servings: 4

Ingredients:
1 green apple, cored and julienned
1 and ½ teaspoons dark sesame oil
4 cups alfalfa sprouts
Salt and black pepper to the taste
1 and ½ teaspoons grape seed oil
¼ cup coconut milk yogurt
4 nasturtium leaves

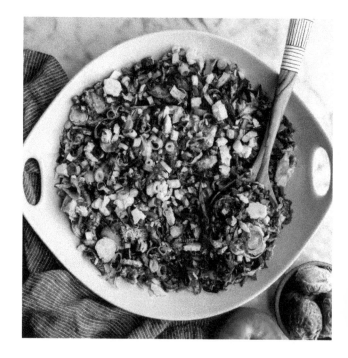

Directions:
1. In a salad bowl mix sprouts with apple and nasturtium.
2. Add salt, pepper, sesame oil, grape seed oil and coconut yogurt, toss to coat and divide between plates.
3. Serve right away.
Enjoy!

Nutrition: calories 100, fat 3, fiber 1, carbs 2, protein 6

Roasted Radishes

Preparation time: 10 minutes
Cooking time: 35 minutes
Servings: 2

Ingredients:
2 cups radishes, cut in quarters
Salt and black pepper to the taste
2 tablespoons ghee, melted
1 tablespoon chives, chopped
1 tablespoon lemon zest

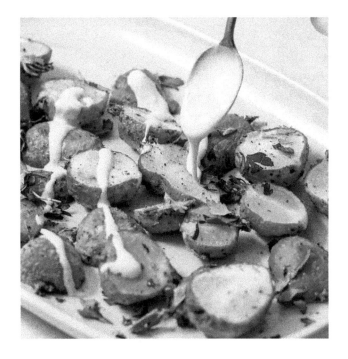

Directions:
1. Spread radishes on a lined baking sheet.
2. Add salt and pepper, chives, lemon zest and ghee, toss to coat and bake in the oven at 375 degrees F for 35 minutes.
3. Divide between plates and serve.
Enjoy!

Nutrition: calories 122, fat 12, fiber 1, carbs 3, protein 14

Radish Hash Browns

Preparation time: 10 minutes
Cooking time: 10 minutes
Servings: 4

Ingredients:
½ teaspoon onion powder
1 pound radishes, shredded
½ teaspoon garlic powder
Salt and black pepper to the taste
4 eggs
1/3 cup parmesan, grated

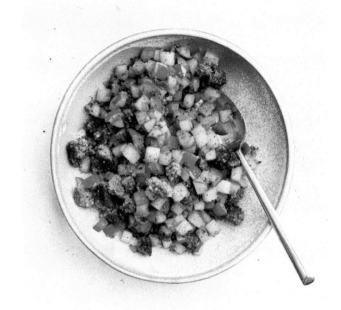

Directions:
1. In a bowl, mix radishes with salt, pepper, onion and garlic powder, eggs and parmesan and stir well.
2. Spread this on a lined baking sheet, introduce in the oven at 375 degrees F and bake for 10 minutes.
3. Divide hash browns between plates and serve.
Enjoy!

Nutrition: calories 80, fat 5, fiber 2, carbs 5, protein 7

Crispy Radishes

Preparation time: 10 minutes
Cooking time: 20 minutes
Servings: 4

Ingredients:
Cooking spray
15 radishes, sliced
Salt and black pepper to the taste
1 tablespoon chives, chopped

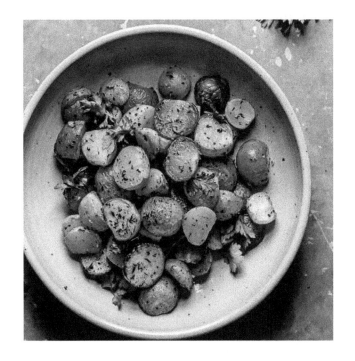

Directions:
1. Arrange radish slices on a lined baking sheet and spray them with cooking oil.
2. Season with salt and pepper and sprinkle chives, introduce in the oven at 375 degrees F and bake for 10 minutes.
3. Flip them and bake for 10 minutes more.
4. Serve them cold.
Enjoy!

Nutrition: calories 30, fat 1, fiber 0.4, carbs 1, protein 0.1

Creamy Radishes

Preparation time: 10 minutes
Cooking time: 25 minutes
Servings: 1

Ingredients:
7 ounces radishes, cut in halves
2 tablespoons sour cream
2 bacon slices
1 tablespoon green onion, chopped
1 tablespoon cheddar cheese, grated
Hot sauce to the taste
Salt and black pepper to the taste

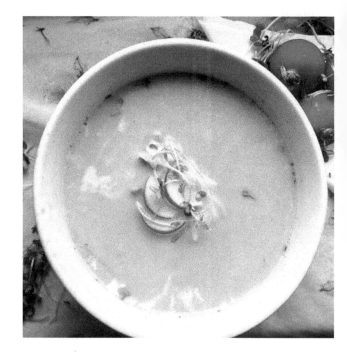

Directions:
1. Put radishes into a pot, add water to cover, bring to a boil over medium heat, cook them for 10 minutes and drain.
2. Heat up a pan over medium high heat, add bacon, cook until it's crispy, transfer to paper towels, drain grease, crumble and leave aside.
3. Return pan to medium heat, add radishes, stir and sauté them for 7 minutes.
4. Add onion, salt, pepper, hot sauce and sour cream, stir and cook for 7 minutes more.
5. Transfer to a plate, top with crumbled bacon and cheddar cheese and serve.
Enjoy!

Nutrition: calories 340, fat 23, fiber 3, carbs 6, protein 15

Radish Soup

Preparation time: 10 minutes
Cooking time: 20 minutes
Servings: 4

Ingredients:
2 bunches radishes, cut in quarters
Salt and black pepper to the taste
6 cups chicken stock
2 stalks celery, chopped
3 tablespoons coconut oil
6 garlic cloves, minced
1 yellow onion, chopped

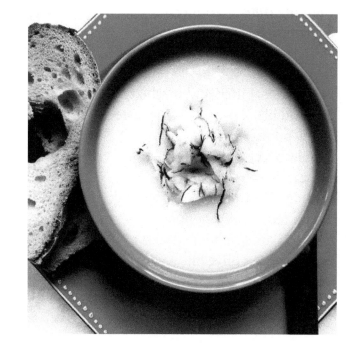

Directions:
1. Heat up a pot with the oil over medium heat, add onion, celery and garlic, stir and cook for 5 minutes.
2. Add radishes, stock, salt and pepper, stir, bring to a boil, cover and simmer for 15 minutes.
3. Divide into soup bowls and serve.
Enjoy!

Nutrition: calories 120, fat 2, fiber 1, carbs 3, protein 10

Tasty Avocado Salad

Preparation time: 10 minutes
Cooking time: 0 minutes
Servings: 4

Ingredients:
2 avocados, pitted and mashed
Salt and black pepper to the taste
¼ teaspoon lemon stevia
1 tablespoon white vinegar
14 ounces coleslaw mix
Juice from 2 limes
¼ cup red onion, chopped
¼ cup cilantro, chopped
2 tablespoons olive oil

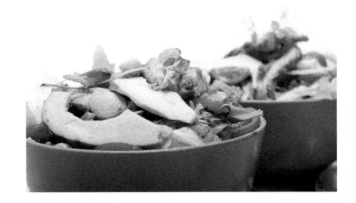

Directions:
1. Put coleslaw mix in a salad bowl. Add avocado mash and onions and toss to coat.
2. In a bowl, mix lime juice with salt, pepper, oil, vinegar and stevia and stir well.
3. Add this to salad, toss to coat, sprinkle cilantro and serve.
Enjoy!

Nutrition: calories 100, fat 10, fiber 2, carbs 5, protein 8

Avocado And Egg Salad

Preparation time: 10 minutes
Cooking time: 7 minutes
Servings: 4

Ingredients:
4 cups mixed lettuce leaves, torn
4 eggs
1 avocado, pitted and sliced
¼ cup mayonnaise
2 teaspoons mustard
2 garlic cloves, minced
1 tablespoon chives, chopped
Salt and black pepper to the taste

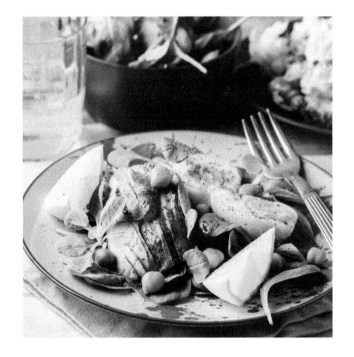

Directions:
1. Put water in a pot, add some salt, add eggs, bring to a boil over medium high heat, boil for 7 minutes, drain, cool, peel and chop them.
2. In a salad bowl, mix lettuce with eggs and avocado.
3. Add chives and garlic, some salt and pepper and toss to coat.
4. In a bowl, mix mustard with mayo, salt and pepper and stir well.
5. Add this to salad, toss well and serve right away.
Enjoy!

Nutrition: calories 234, fat 12, fiber 4, carbs 7, protein 12

Avocado And Cucumber Salad

Preparation time: 10 minutes
Cooking time: 0 minutes
Servings: 4

Ingredients:
1 small red onion, sliced
1 cucumber, sliced
2 avocados, pitted, peeled and chopped
1 pound cherry tomatoes, halved
2 tablespoons olive oil
¼ cup cilantro, chopped
2 tablespoons lemon juice
Salt and black pepper to the taste

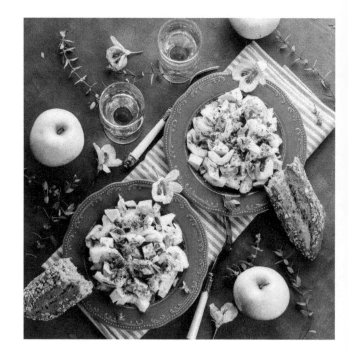

Directions:
1. In a large salad bowl, mix tomatoes with cucumber, onion and avocado and stir.
2. Add oil, salt, pepper and lemon juice and toss to coat well.
3. Serve cold with cilantro on top.
Enjoy!

Nutrition: calories 140, fat 4, fiber 2, carbs 4, protein 5

Delicious Avocado Soup

Preparation time: 10 minutes
Cooking time: 10 minutes
Servings: 4

Ingredients:
2 avocados, pitted, peeled and chopped
3 cups chicken stock
2 scallions, chopped
Salt and black pepper to the taste
2 tablespoons ghee
2/3 cup heavy cream

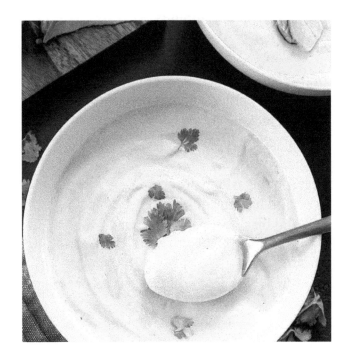

Directions:
1. Heat up a pot with the ghee over medium heat, add scallions, stir and cook for 2 minutes.
2. Add 2 and ½ cups stock, stir and simmer for 3 minutes.
3. In your blender, mix avocados with the rest of the stock, salt, pepper and heavy cream and pulse well.
4. Add this to the pot, stir well, cook for 2 minutes and season with more salt and pepper.
5. Stir well, ladle into soup bowls and serve.
Enjoy!

Nutrition: calories 332, fat 23, fiber 4, carbs 6, protein 6

Delicious Avocado And Bacon Soup

Preparation time: 10 minutes
Cooking time: 10 minutes
Servings: 4

Ingredients:
2 avocados, pitted and cut in halves
4 cups chicken stock
1/3 cup cilantro, chopped
Juice of ½ lime
1 teaspoon garlic powder
½ pound bacon, cooked and chopped
Salt and black pepper to the taste

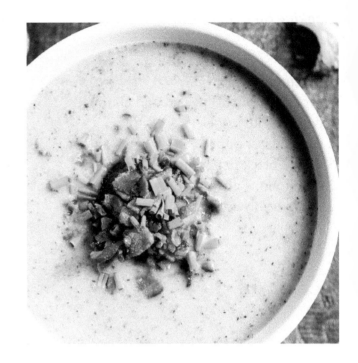

Directions:
1. Put stock in a pot and bring to a boil over medium high heat.
2. In your blender, mix avocados with garlic powder, cilantro, lime juice, salt and pepper and blend well.
3. Add this to stock and blend using an immersion blender.
4. Add bacon, more salt and pepper the taste, stir, cook for 3 minutes, ladle into soup bowls and serve.
Enjoy!

Nutrition: calories 300, fat 23, fiber 5, carbs 6, protein 17

Thai Avocado Soup

Preparation time: 10 minutes
Cooking time: 10 minutes
Servings: 4

Ingredients:
1 cup coconut milk
2 teaspoons Thai green curry paste
1 avocado, pitted, peeled and chopped
1 tablespoon cilantro, chopped
Salt and black pepper to the taste
2 cups veggie stock
Lime wedges for serving

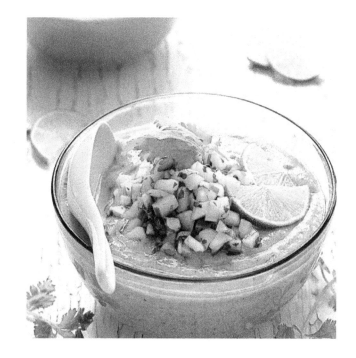

Directions:
1. In your blender, mix avocado with salt, pepper, curry paste and coconut milk and pulse well.
2. Transfer this to a pot and heat up over medium heat.
3. Add stock, stir, bring to a simmer and cook for 5 minutes.
4. Add cilantro, more salt and pepper, stir, cook for 1 minute more, ladle into soup bowls and serve with lime wedges on the side.
Enjoy!

Nutrition: calories 240, fat 4, fiber 2, carbs 6, protein 12

Simple Arugula Salad

Preparation time: 10 minutes
Cooking time: 0 minutes
Servings: 4

Ingredients:
1 white onion, chopped
1 tablespoon vinegar
1 cup hot water
1 bunch baby arugula
¼ cup walnuts, chopped
2 tablespoons cilantro, chopped
2 garlic cloves, minced
2 tablespoons olive oil
Salt and black pepper to the taste
1 tablespoon lemon juice

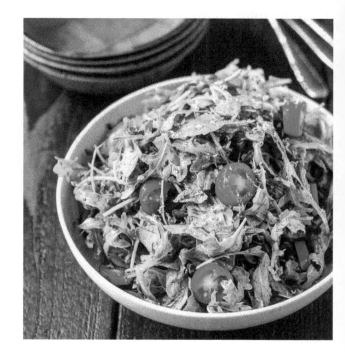

Directions:
1. In a bowl, mix water with vinegar, add onion, leave aside for 5 minutes, drain well and press.
2. In a salad bowl, mix arugula with walnuts and onion and stir.
3. Add garlic, salt, pepper, lemon juice, cilantro and oil, toss well and serve.
Enjoy!

Nutrition: calories 200, fat 2, fiber 1, carbs 5, protein 7

Arugula Soup

Preparation time: 10 minutes
Cooking time: 13 minutes
Servings: 6

Ingredients:
1 yellow onion, chopped
1 tablespoon olive oil
2 garlic cloves, minced
½ cup coconut milk
10 ounces baby arugula
¼ cup mixed mint, tarragon and parsley
2 tablespoons chives, chopped
4 tablespoons coconut milk yogurt
6 cups chicken stock
Salt and black pepper to the taste

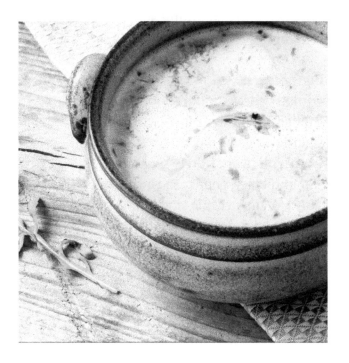

Directions:
1. Heat up a pot with the oil over medium high heat, add onion and garlic, stir and cook for 5 minutes.
2. Add stock and milk, stir and bring to a simmer.
3. Add arugula, tarragon, parsley and mint, stir and cook everything for 6 minutes.
4. Add coconut yogurt, salt, pepper and chives, stir, cook for 2 minutes, divide into soup bowls and serve.
Enjoy!

Nutrition: calories 200, fat 4, fiber 2, carbs 6, protein 10

Arugula And Broccoli Soup

Preparation time: 10 minutes
Cooking time: 20 minutes
Servings: 4

Ingredients:
1 small yellow onion, chopped
1 tablespoon olive oil
1 garlic clove, minced
1 broccoli head, florets separated
Salt and black pepper to the taste
2 and ½ cups veggie stock
1 teaspoon cumin, ground
Juice of ½ lemon
1 cup arugula leaves

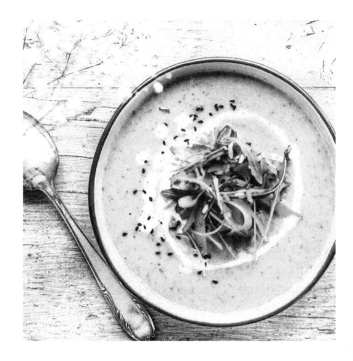

Directions:
1. Heat up a pot with the oil over medium high heat, add onions, stir and cook for 4 minutes.
2. Add garlic, stir and cook for 1 minute.
3. Add broccoli, cumin, salt and pepper, stir and cook for 4 minutes.
4. Add stock, stir and cook for 8 minutes.
5. Blend soup using an immersion blender, add half of the arugula and blend again.
6. Add the rest of the arugula, stir and heat up the soup again.
7. Add lemon juice, stir, ladle into soup bowls and serve.
Enjoy!

Nutrition: calories 150, fat 3, fiber 1, carbs 3, protein 7

Delicious Zucchini Cream

Preparation time: 10 minutes
Cooking time: 25 minutes
Servings: 8

Ingredients:
6 zucchinis, cut in halves and then sliced
Salt and black pepper to the taste
1 tablespoon ghee
28 ounces veggie stock
1 teaspoon oregano, dried
½ cup yellow onion, chopped
3 garlic cloves, minced
2 ounces parmesan, grated
¾ cup heavy cream

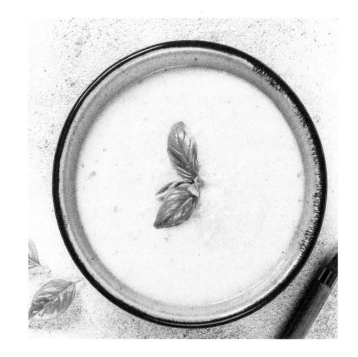

Directions:
1. Heat up a pot with the ghee over medium high heat, add onion, stir and cook for 4 minutes.
2. Add garlic, stir and cook for 2 minutes more.
3. Add zucchinis, stir and cook for 3 minutes.
4. Add stock, stir, bring to a boil and simmer over medium heat for 15 minutes.
5. Add oregano, salt and pepper, stir, take off heat and blend using an immersion blender.
6. Heat up soup again, add heavy cream, stir and bring to a simmer.
7. Add parmesan, stir, take off heat, ladle into bowls and serve right away.
Enjoy!

Nutrition: calories 160, fat 4, fiber 2, carbs 4, protein 8

Zucchini And Avocado Soup

Preparation time: 10 minutes
Cooking time: 15 minutes
Servings: 4

Ingredients:
1 big avocado, pitted, peeled and chopped
4 scallions, chopped
1 teaspoon ginger, grated
2 tablespoons avocado oil
Salt and black pepper to the taste
2 zucchinis, chopped
29 ounces veggie stock
1 garlic clove, minced
1 cup water
1 tablespoon lemon juice
1 red bell pepper, chopped

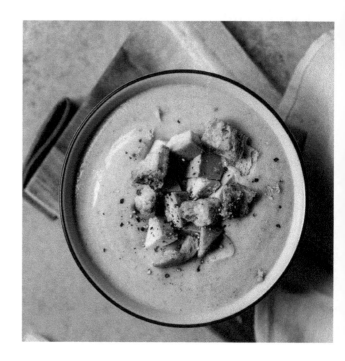

Directions:
1. Heat up a pot with the oil over medium heat, add onions, stir and cook for 3 minutes.
2. Add garlic and ginger, stir and cook for 1 minute.
3. Add zucchini, salt, pepper, water and stock, stir, bring to a boil, cover pot and cook for 10 minutes.
4. Take off heat, leave soup aside for a couple of minutes, add avocado, stir, blend everything using an immersion blender and heat up again.
5. Add more salt and pepper, bell pepper and lemon juice, stir, heat up soup again, ladle into soup bowls and serve.
Enjoy!

Nutrition: calories 154, fat 12, fiber 3, carbs 5, protein 4

Swiss Chard Pie

Preparation time: 10 minutes
Cooking time: 45 minutes
Servings: 12

Ingredients:
8 cups Swiss chard, chopped
½ cup onion, chopped
1 tablespoon olive oil
1 garlic clove, minced
Salt and black pepper to the taste
3 eggs
2 cups ricotta cheese
1 cup mozzarella, shredded
A pinch of nutmeg
¼ cup parmesan, grated
1 pound sausage, chopped

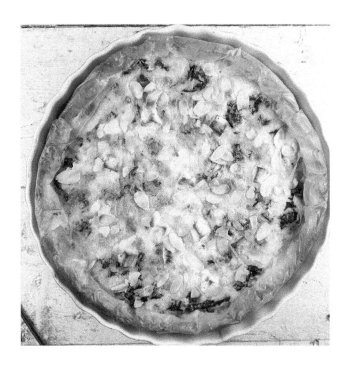

Directions:
1. Heat up a pan with the oil over medium heat, add onions and garlic, stir and cook for 3 minutes.
2. Add Swiss chard, stir and cook for 5 minutes more.
3. Add salt, pepper and nutmeg, stir, take off heat and leave aside for a few minutes.
4. In a bowl, whisk eggs with mozzarella, parmesan and ricotta and stir well.
5. Add Swiss chard mix and stir well.
6. Spread sausage meat on the bottom of a pie pan and press well.
7. Add Swiss chard and eggs mix, spread well, introduce in the oven at 350 degrees F and bake for 35 minutes.
8. Leave pie aside to cool down, slice and serve it.
Enjoy!

Nutrition: calories 332, fat 23, fiber 3, carbs 4, protein 23

Swiss Chard Salad

Preparation time: 10 minutes
Cooking time: 20 minutes
Servings: 4

Ingredients:
1 bunch Swiss chard, cut into strips
2 tablespoons avocado oil
1 small yellow onion, chopped
A pinch of red pepper flakes
¼ cup pine nuts, toasted
¼ cup raisins
1 tablespoon balsamic vinegar
Salt and black pepper to the taste

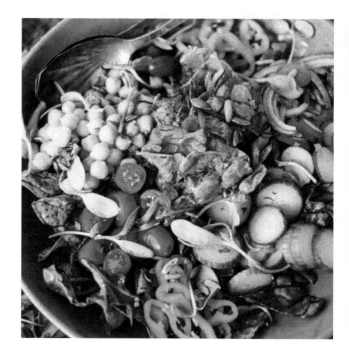

Directions:
1. Heat up a pan with the oil over medium heat, add chard and onions, stir and cook for 5 minutes.
2. Add salt, pepper and pepper flakes, stir and cook for 3 minutes more.
3. Put raisins in a bowl, add water to cover them, heat them up in your microwave for 1 minute, leave aside for 5 minutes and drain them well.
4. Add raisins and pine nuts to the pan, also add vinegar, stir, cook for 3 minutes more, divide between plates and serve.
Enjoy!

Nutrition: calories 120, fat 2, fiber 1, carbs 4, protein 8

Green Salad

Preparation time: 10 minutes
Cooking time: 0 minutes
Servings: 4

Ingredients:
4 handfuls grapes, halved
1 bunch Swiss chard, chopped
1 avocado, pitted, peeled and cubed
Salt and black pepper to the taste
2 tablespoons avocado oil
1 tablespoon mustard
7 sage leaves, chopped
1 garlic clove, minced

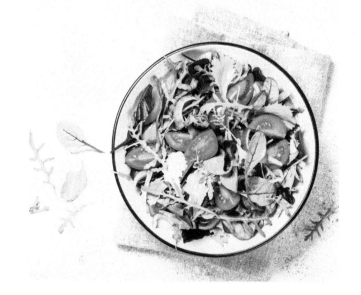

Directions:
1. In a salad bowl, mix Swiss chard with grapes and avocado cubes.
2. In a bowl, mix mustard with oil, sage, garlic, salt and pepper and whisk well.
3. Add this to salad, toss to coat well and serve.
Enjoy!

Nutrition: calories 120, fat 2, fiber 1, carbs 4, protein 5

Catalan Style Greens

Preparation time: 10 minutes
Cooking time: 15 minutes
Servings: 4

Ingredients:
1 apple, cored and chopped
1 yellow onion, sliced
3 tablespoons avocado oil
¼ cup raisins
6 garlic cloves, chopped
¼ cup pine nuts, toasted
¼ cup balsamic vinegar
5 cups mixed spinach and chard
Salt and black pepper to the taste
A pinch of nutmeg

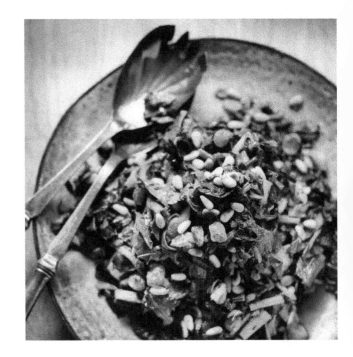

Directions:
1. Heat up a pan with the oil over medium high heat, add onion, stir and cook for 3 minutes.
2. Add apple, stir and cook for 4 minutes more.
3. Add garlic, stir and cook for 1 minute.
4. Add raisins, vinegar and mixed spinach and chard, stir and cook for 5 minutes.
5. Add nutmeg, salt and pepper, stir, cook for a few seconds more, divide between plates and serve.
Enjoy!

Nutrition: calories 120, fat 1, fiber 2, carbs 3, protein 6

Swiss Chard Soup

Preparation time: 10 minutes
Cooking time: 35 minutes
Servings: 12

Ingredients:
4 cups Swiss chard, chopped
4 cups chicken breast, cooked and shredded
2 cups water
1 cup mushrooms, sliced
1 tablespoon garlic, minced
1 tablespoon coconut oil, melted
¼ cup onion, chopped
8 cups chicken stock
2 cups yellow squash, chopped
1 cup green beans, cut into medium pieces
2 tablespoons vinegar
¼ cup basil, chopped
Salt and black pepper to the taste
4 bacon slices, chopped
¼ cup sundried tomatoes, chopped

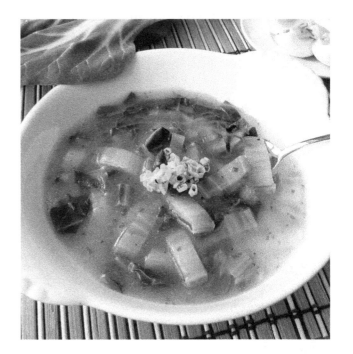

Directions:
1. Heat up a pot with the oil over medium high heat, add bacon, stir and cook for 2 minutes. Add tomatoes, garlic, onions and mushrooms, stir and cook for 5 minutes.
2. Add water, stock and chicken, stir and cook for 15 minutes.
3. Add Swiss chard, green beans, squash, salt and pepper, stir and cook for 10 minutes more.
4. Add vinegar, basil, more salt and pepper if needed, stir, ladle into soup bowls and serve. Enjoy!

Nutrition: calories 140, fat 4, fiber 2, carbs 4, protein 18

Special Swiss Chard Soup

Preparation time: 10 minutes
Cooking time: 2 hours and 10 minutes
Servings: 4

Ingredients:
1 red onion, chopped
1 bunch Swiss chard, chopped
1 yellow squash, chopped
1 zucchini, chopped
1 green bell pepper, chopped
Salt and black pepper to the taste
6 carrots, chopped
4 cups tomatoes, chopped
1 cup cauliflower florets, chopped
1 cup green beans, chopped
6 cups chicken stock
7 ounces canned tomato paste
2 cups water
1 pound sausage, chopped
2 garlic cloves, minced
2 teaspoons thyme, chopped
1 teaspoon rosemary, dried
1 tablespoon fennel, minced
½ teaspoon red pepper flakes
Some grated parmesan for serving

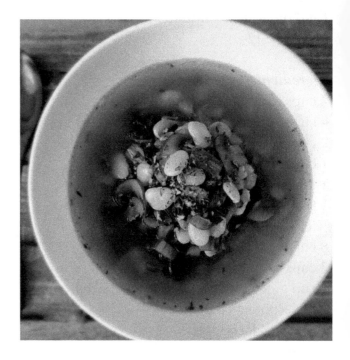

Directions:
1. Heat up a pan over medium high heat, add sausage and garlic, stir and cook until it browns and transfer along with its juices to your slow cooker.
2. Add onion, Swiss chard, squash, bell pepper, zucchini, carrots, tomatoes, cauliflower, green beans, tomato paste, stock, water, thyme, fennel, rosemary, pepper flakes, salt and pepper, stir, cover and cook on High for 2 hours.
3. Uncover pot, stir soup, ladle into bowls, sprinkle parmesan on top and serve.
Enjoy!

Nutrition: calories 150, fat 8, fiber 2, carbs 4, protein 9

Roasted Tomato Cream

Preparation time: 10 minutes
Cooking time: 1 hour
Servings: 8

Ingredients:
1 jalapeno pepper, chopped
4 garlic cloves, minced
2 pounds cherry tomatoes, cut in halves
1 yellow onion, cut into wedges
Salt and black pepper to the taste
¼ cup olive oil
½ teaspoon oregano, dried
4 cups chicken stock
¼ cup basil, chopped
½ cup parmesan, grated

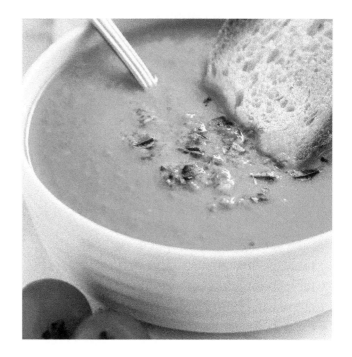

Directions:
1. Spread tomatoes and onion in a baking dish. Add garlic and chili pepper, season with salt, pepper and oregano and drizzle the oil.
2. Toss to coat and bake in the oven at 425 degrees F for 30 minutes.
3. Take tomatoes mix out of the oven, transfer to a pot, add stock
and heat everything up over medium high heat. 4. Bring to a boil, cover pot, reduce heat and simmer for 20 minutes.
5. Blend using an immersion blender, add salt and pepper to the taste and basil, stir and ladle into soup bowls.
6. Sprinkle parmesan on top and serve.
Enjoy!

Nutrition: calories 140, fat 2, fiber 2, carbs 5, protein 8

Eggplant Soup

Preparation time: 10 minutes
Cooking time: 50 minutes
Servings: 4

Ingredients:
4 tomatoes
1 teaspoon garlic, minced
¼ yellow onion, chopped
Salt and black pepper to the taste
2 cups chicken stock
1 bay leaf
½ cup heavy cream
2 tablespoons basil, chopped
4 tablespoons parmesan, grated
1 tablespoon olive oil
1 eggplant, chopped

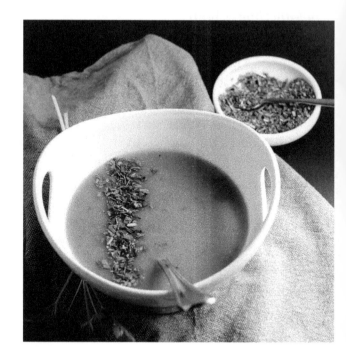

Directions:
1. Spread eggplant pieces on a baking sheet, mix with oil, onion, garlic, salt and pepper, introduce in the oven at 400 degrees F and bake for 15 minutes.
2. Put water in a pot, bring to a boil over medium heat, add tomatoes, steam them for 1 minutes, peel them and chop.
3. Take eggplant mix out of the oven and transfer to a pot.
4. Add tomatoes, stock, bay leaf, salt and pepper, stir, bring to a boil and simmer for 30 minutes.
5. Add heavy cream, basil and parmesan, stir, ladle into soup bowls and serve.
Enjoy!

Nutrition: calories 180, fat 2, fiber 3, carbs 5, protein 10

Eggplant Stew

Preparation time: 10 minutes
Cooking time: 30 minutes
Servings: 4

Ingredients:
1 red onion, chopped
2 garlic cloves, chopped
1 bunch parsley, chopped
Salt and black pepper to the taste
1 teaspoon oregano, dried
2 eggplants, cut into medium chunks
2 tablespoons olive oil
2 tablespoons capers, chopped
1 handful green olives, pitted and sliced
5 tomatoes, chopped
3 tablespoons herb vinegar

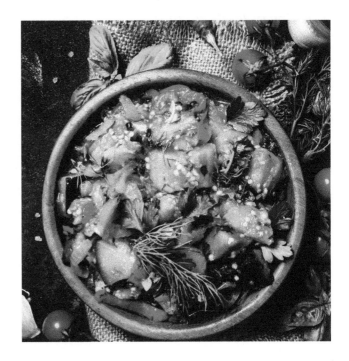

Directions:
1. Heat up a pot with the oil over medium heat, add eggplant, oregano, salt and pepper, stir and cook for 5 minutes.
2. Add garlic, onion and parsley, stir and cook for 4 minutes.
3. Add capers, olives, vinegar and tomatoes, stir and cook for 15 minutes.
4. Add more salt and pepper if needed, stir, divide into bowls and serve.
Enjoy!

Nutrition: calories 200, fat 13, fiber 3, carbs 5, protein 7

Roasted Bell Peppers Soup

Preparation time: 10 minutes
Cooking time: 15 minutes
Servings: 6

Ingredients:
12 ounces roasted bell peppers, chopped
2 tablespoons olive oil
2 garlic cloves, minced
29 ounces canned chicken stock
Salt and black pepper to the taste
7 ounces water
2/3 cup heavy cream
1 yellow onion, chopped
¼ cup parmesan, grated
2 celery stalks, chopped

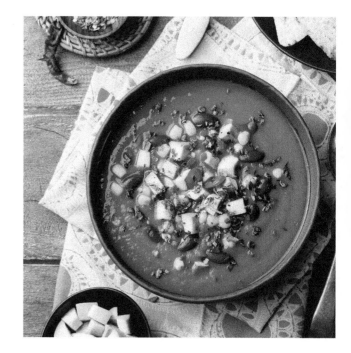

Directions:
1. Heat up a pot with the oil over medium heat, add onion, garlic, celery, some salt and pepper, stir and cook for 8 minutes.
2. Add bell peppers, water and stock, stir, bring to a boil, cover, reduce heat and simmer for 5 minutes.
3. Use an immersion blender to puree the soup, then add more salt, pepper and cream, stir, bring to a boil and take off heat.
4. Ladle into bowls, sprinkle parmesan and serve.
Enjoy!

Nutrition: calories 176, fat 13, fiber 1, carbs 4, protein 6

9 781803 211008